Welcome to Critical Anatomy. The name of this book is inte.

In a study published in 2016, Yoga Journal and Yoga Alliance found that the number of yoga practitioners increased by 50 percent since 2012 - to over 36 million people in just the United States alone.

There are currently two people interested in becoming a yoga teacher for every one existing yoga teacher.

This increase in participants and in newly trained yoga teachers has also seen an increase in yoga injury, unfortunately. A recent study found that more than one in every ten participants experienced musculoskeletal pain - which is comparable to the rate of injuries from all other sports. This is up to 10 times higher than previously thought. To add, yoga can also exacerbate existing injury and pain, with over 20 percent of existing injuries made worse by doing yoga.

The good news is that we have the power to change these statistics going forward. By educating ourselves, educating current instructors, and educating future instructors we can build the body of knowledge that is required to prevent injury. We also allow ourselves to pass this knowledge onto the students themselves.

Not only is anatomy knowledge useful, but it is critical to improving the yoga industry.

This book is designed to be a reference for you, as the practicing yogi or the yoga instructor. For your own teaching or as a reference during a teacher training program for anatomy and physiology education of teacher trainees.

Appendix A is a separate manual that is for teacher trainees to use as a workbook during their teacher training. They can then keep this workbook for future reference in their teaching.

This book covers:
- Systems of the body: skeletal, muscular, cardiovascular, respiratory, endocrine, and digestive.
- Common yoga injuries, their causes, prevention, and impact on yoga.
- Breakdown and assessment of alignment and anatomy/physiology principles in many of the key yoga postures across all groups of yoga asana.

The manual includes:
- An outline for teacher trainees to fill in during your anatomy and physiology lectures.
- A competency quiz for your trainees to complete at the end of their anatomy section of teacher training.

The information within this handbook (and the corresponding workbook) not only meets, but exceeds, requirements by Yoga Alliance for 200 hour teacher trainings.

You ARE NOT permitted to reproduce any part of this book. You are permitted to make copies of the manual only for your teacher trainees to use and keep.

All photos are courtesy of Tony Brand and all diagrams and images are reproduced and published with permission of and licensed from Pond5.com.

Why do we study anatomy?

Yoga is a spiritual practice, it's an energetic practice, it's a mental practice, but it is also a physical practice. As a yoga teacher you are responsible for taking many different physical bodies through postures, poses, and transitions that are meant to stretch and strengthen different structures in the body. As a yoga practitioner, you are responsible for taking your own body through these postures. Like any other physical practice, there is an opportunity for injury to occur during yoga. As a teacher, you will also be teaching to a variety of body types, pre-existing injuries or conditions, and ages. Having an understanding of human anatomy and mechanics allows you to intelligently plan and sequence classes, cue (verbally and physically) people into and out of postures, prevent pain and injury, and assist yourself or students in safely modifying their practices.

Yoga traditionally was practiced by boys and young men starting from a very young age. The functional anatomy and physiology of these students is undoubtedly different than the functional anatomy and physiology of a modern day yoga student. Modern day students live and work in a culture that is much more sedentary and sitting focused than ever before. Most modern day students didn't (or won't) begin a yoga practice until much later in their lives. These two factors mean that understanding anatomy, not just memorizing postures and cues, is essential for safely teaching and practicing yoga.

Completing this manual (and the associated in person training, if you choose to take it) does not give you a medical degree of any sort. It does not give you the knowledge or legal ability to diagnose or treat your students, but it does give you the information to be the smartest yoga instructor you can be.

Systems of the Body

The body is organized into systems. Each system has a particular function and purpose in the human body, but they are not independent of each other. They work interdependently to maintain homeostasis and equilibrium in the body and to adapt to the changing environments both inside and outside the body.

System Overview:

- **Muscular**: The muscular system is an organ system consisting of skeletal, smooth and cardiac muscles. It permits movement of the body, maintains posture, and circulates blood throughout the body. The focus of our study on the muscular system is on skeletal muscles (those that attach to the skeleton). Smooth muscles make up our internal organs and cardiac muscles are the muscles of the heart.

- **Skeletal**: The skeletal system is the framework of the body, consisting of bones and other connective tissues, which protects and supports the body tissues and internal organs. The skeleton can be split into two sections: axial and appendicular. The axial skeleton is the skull and bones of the spine (vertebrae) while the appendicular skeleton are the bones of both the upper and lower extremities. Other connective tissues in the body include tendons (the attachments between muscles and bones), ligaments (they connect bones to other bones), and cartilage (a shock absorber found in joints).

- **Nervous**: The nervous system consists of the brain and the network of nerve cells and fibers. The nervous system is responsible for carrying signals from the brain to other parts of the body (to create movement, for example) as well as taking information from the body back to the brain (about external conditions, like temperature, as an example). The nervous system has three parts: the central nervous system (the brain and spinal cord), the peripheral nervous system (the nerves that take information from the spinal cord to the body and vice versa), and the autonomic nervous system (comprised of the sympathetic and parasympathetic systems, which regulate much of the body's function).

- **Cardiovascular**: This system's function is the interaction of the heart and blood vessels as they work to circulate blood throughout the body. The two main types of blood vessels are arteries and veins. Arteries carry fresh oxygen to the body, while veins carry waste products via the bloodstream back to the lungs to exchange and replenish the body's oxygen supply.

- **Respiratory:** The respiratory system is the system of breathing. Consisting of the trachea (windpipe), bronchi, and lungs the main function of the respiratory system is to inhale oxygen and exhale waste product such as carbon dioxide. This system works very closely with the cardiovascular system.

- **Digestive:** The digestive system is comprised of the organs of digestion and elimination, following the path of food from the time it enters the body until the time it leaves the body. The digestive system is managed with a combination of input from the nervous system, the endocrine system, and the muscular system. Yoga and meditation as a practice can have an effect on the functioning of the digestive system.

- **Endocrine:** The endocrine system includes the hormone system of the body as well as the glands that release hormones. Hormones act as controls for many of the other body systems. The functioning of the endocrine system controls everything from mood to digestion to heart rate. You will learn how different aspects of yoga and yoga postures impact the endocrine system.

Teaching Takeaways:
- The body is organized into systems by function.
- Systems do not work independently of one another.
- This and the 200 hour teacher training anatomy guide are an overview of anatomy. You (and your students) are encouraged to continue your studies if anatomy is an area of yoga that is of interest.

Let's begin our anatomy journey by taking an in depth look at each system individually.

Muscular System:

As we noted above, of the three types of muscles in the body, yogis primarily focus on the skeletal muscles. There are approximately 650 skeletal muscles in the body. As a yoga instructor it is not imperative to know each and every muscle, but an understanding of specific muscles will enhance your ability to teach yoga safely and effectively.

First, let's look at the anatomy of a muscle. Muscle fibers are aligned similarly to telephone or electrical cables. Groups of fibers are bound into small bundles, those small bundles are collected and bound into larger bundles, etc. Fibers in healthy muscles all run the same direction, which gives them ability to contract as well as to be stretched or lengthened. After injury, muscle fibers can be repaired with scar tissue which doesn't necessarily realign itself the same way as the rest of the muscle. This causes potential weaknesses and imperfections in the muscle tissue. Care should be taken with stretching previously injured muscles to avoid re-tearing them.

The function of the muscular system is to create motion and to provide support to the skeleton against gravity.

As mentioned earlier, while you don't need to know every muscle, there are important muscles to know. We will explore these muscles and their function during yoga by breaking the body into different parts.

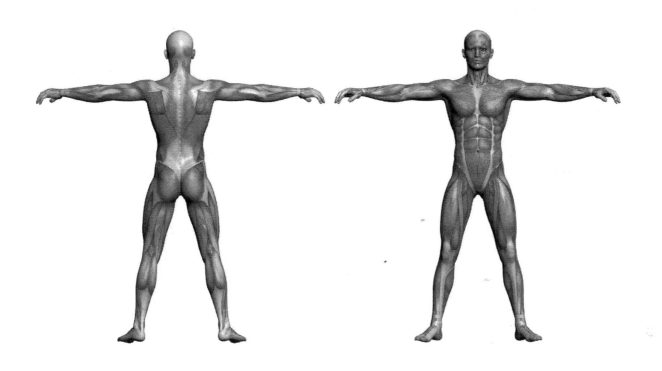

- Trapezius
- Rhomboids
- Erector Spinae
- Latissimus Dorsi
- Rectus Abdominis
- Obliques
- Transverse Abdominis
- Gluteus Maximus
- Gluteus Medius
- Psoas
- Quadriceps
- Hamstrings
- Pectoralis
- Deltoid
- Rotator Cuff

- **The Back**:
  1. Trapezius: This muscle runs from the base of the skull (occiput) to the shoulder blade (scapula) and attaches to the spine along the cervical and thoracic vertebrae. We primarily see the function of its upper fibers by causing the shoulders to shrug towards the ears when the muscle is contracted or shortened. In many people, this portion of the muscle is chronically shortened due to postural changes related to sitting (during driving, at a computer, on cell phones, etc). Often in yoga our focus is on relaxing or lengthening the trapezius to allow the shoulders to move down the back and the neck to lengthen.

  2. Rhomboids: This muscle group lies between the shoulder blades (scapula) and the spine. When contracted it draws the shoulder blades towards each other (retraction). Rhomboids are essential in upright posture. Often these muscles are underdeveloped due to the rounded upper back/shoulder posture associated with sitting. Postures like airplane arms, cobra, and locust are excellent for building strength and endurance in the rhomboids.

  3. Erector spinae: The erector muscles run longitudinally from the base of the skull to the base of the spine. Their purpose is to help hold the spine upright (or erect). Again, they are postural muscles but also play a role in core stability. Locust, bow, and warrior three are all excellent postures for strengthening the erectors.

  4. Latissimus Dorsi: The latissimus dorsi are two of the largest muscles in the body (in terms of surface area). They cover the majority of the posterior trunk and are responsible for upright posture as well as shoulder extension. They must be opened in order to proper work into postures such as wheel and they are very active in all arm balances and inversions.

- **Abdominal musculature:**

  1. Rectus abdominis: These muscles are commonly known as the "six-pack" muscles. They lie on the anterior (front) wall of the torso and cause flexion of the spine (drawing the ribs toward the pelvis, such as in a sit-up) when contracted. While they are excellent "mover" muscles, they play a much smaller role in stability compared to other core muscles. Plank and boat pose are useful for strengthening the rectus.

  2. Obliques: The obliques lie on the lateral (side) walls of the torso and are responsible for the motions of side bending and rotation. Along with the

8

transverse abdominis, the rectus abdominis, and the erector spinae, the obliques help create a corset-like stabilizer for the abdomen and lumbar spine. Side plank is a good choice for oblique strengthening.

3. Transverse abdominis: This muscle lies deep to the rectus and obliques and runs perpendicular to the rectus. This gives it the action of drawing the abdominal wall inward when contracted. This muscle is a stabilizer and is built for endurance. A properly functioning transverse abdominis will create stability through the torso and protect the low back. It will also provide a stable base for upper and lower body muscles during movement. Unfortunately this muscle is often under conditioned. The action of drawing the low belly up and in towards the spine (known as uddiyana bandha) activates the transverse abdominis.

- **Posterior Hips:**

1. Gluteus maximus: This is the largest of the glute muscle group and is the one people think of most often. The gluteus maximus is primarily responsible for extension of the hip. Despite being one of the largest muscle groups in the body, it tends to be underdeveloped due to the long periods of time spent sitting. Poses to strengthen the glutes include bridges as well as any lunge or squat posture if the weight is placed into the heels (versus the balls) of the feet.

2. Gluteus medius: The middle sized glute muscle lies on the outer hip and is an important stabilizer, especially while in single leg standing (most balance postures). A strong gluteus medius will keep the pelvis level and the joints of the lower extremity stacked, thereby providing injury protection. In general, women have wider hips than men. This difference in angle causes more weakness in the gluteus medius in women. Weakness plus the resulting angle at the knee can result in knee injuries in women. Therefore, strengthening the gluteus medius in women is especially important. Side plank as well as most standing balance postures will help build strength here.

- **Hip Flexors:**

1. Psoas: The iliopsoas is the muscle group commonly known as hip flexors. When engaged they close the angle between the torso and the thigh, by either bringing the knee into the chest or folding the torso forward (depending on positioning). The psoas is the more important muscle of the two as it has direct attachment from the leg (via the femur/thigh bone) to the spine (via the lumbar vertebrae). This means that tightness in the psoas can influence not only hip position, but also pelvis and low back position. Many students will have tightness in their hip flexors, once again

9

poses
bridge } weight
lunge }   ↓
squat } heel

*poses
- standing balance
- side plank

PSOAJ
femur →
lumbar
vertebrae

poses
low lunge
modified
crescent
*stabilize llow
back

due to the predominance of sitting in our culture. In many yoga postures we aim to lengthen the psoas, however it should be noted that in order to truly stretch the hip flexor, the lumbar spine needs to be stabilized (via activation of the transverse abdominis). With that stabilization, poses such as low lunge or modified crescent are excellent psoas lengtheners.

uddiyana [handwritten]

- **Quadriceps:**
  1. "Quad" is Latin for "four" and describes the number of muscles that make up the quadriceps. This muscle group lies on the anterior (front) of the thigh and is responsible for two actions: extending/straightening the knee and assisting with flexion of the hip. The quadriceps are very often used in yoga postures. They are active during all warrior stances, chair pose, and even tadasana. Most people exhibit increased tightness and over activity of the quads compared to the muscles of the posterior thigh (like the hamstrings). A well rounded yoga practice should include opening of the quadriceps with poses such as low lunge, dancers, or bow. This will help with alignment in backbending postures as well.

*poses
low lunge } open
dancer }
bow
warrior } strengthen
chair* [handwritten]

- **Hamstrings:**
  1. The hamstrings are a group of three muscles that lie on the posterior (back) aspect of the thigh. The hamstrings are primarily responsible for flexion (bending) of the knee. The hamstrings should be between 60-75% of the strength of the quadriceps. Because they tend to be weaker than that, they have to work harder to balance out the strength of the quadriceps in daily activities (as well as yoga postures). This can result in tightness of the hamstrings as well as overuse. Bridge pose is an excellent hamstring strengthening posture. Cuing students to shift weight into their heels in standing postures will also encourage hamstring activation.

*poses
- bridge (heels) for strength
- folds for flex* [handwritten]

- **Upper Body:**
  1. **Pectoralis:** The main muscle group of the anterior chest wall is the pectoralis. The pectoralis group consists of two muscles: the pectoralis major and the pectoralis minor. Both muscles contribute to postural malalignment when they are shortened or tight (often due to prolonged sitting or computer use). Opening the chest musculature with yoga postures can help with creating space and opportunity to strengthen the upper back muscles. The shoulder blades cannot draw towards each other or improve strength in the rhomboids without the chest being open. An open chest also plays a role in lung capacity and the ability to breathe deeply. Postures that are good for opening the chest include wide baby cobra, anuvittasana (cactus arms), and interlacing the hands behind the low back.

*Open pectoralis
- wide baby cobra
- cactus arms
- interlaced hands* [handwritten]

poses
in 11

poses
hands on ground
-plank
-DD
-UD

2. **Deltoid:** The deltoid is a large shoulder muscle that lies on the superior and lateral aspect of the shoulder (think of it as being where a shoulder pad would be). It is responsible for abducting (moving the arm outward), flexing the arm overhead, as well as playing a role in extension (bringing the arm behind the low back). Extended arms in Warrior 2 will help strengthen the deltoid.

3. **Rotator cuff:** The rotator cuff is a group of four small muscles that surround the glenohumeral (shoulder) joint. Individually, they each play a role in rotation of the humerus (upper arm bone) either internally or externally. As a group, their job is to stabilize the shoulder joint and keep the ball in the socket. The shoulder joint is inherently unstable, and trades that stability for a larger range of motion (allowing us to reach overhead, behind our backs, etc.). It relies on the rotator cuff for it's dynamic stability and protection. Postures where the hands are planted on the ground (plank, downward facing dog, upward facing dog) are great rotator cuff stabilizers. The rotator cuff is easily injured in yoga due to excess stress placed on the small muscles and improper alignment in poses such as chaturanga.

This has been an incredibly brief overview of the muscular system. The goal of this review is to inform the student of some of the major movers of the body that we experience and interact with in yoga postures. This is far from a comprehensive list and many other muscles have large roles to play.

Skeletal System:

The adult human body has 206 bones that create it's skeleton. The skeleton can be separated into two pieces, the axial skeleton (skull and spine) and the appendicular skeleton (the extremities). The skeleton is a support system for the body, protection for vital organs, and attachment points for muscles to create levers and allow for movement.

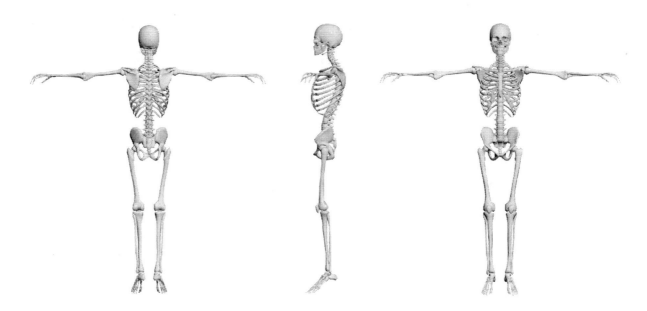

Regions of the body:
- **Spine:**

Human vertebral column

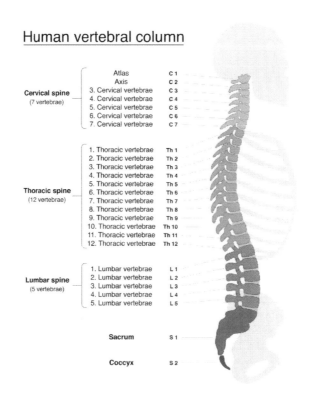

Cervical spine (7 vertebrae)	Atlas	C 1
	Axis	C 2
	3. Cervical vertebrae	C 3
	4. Cervical vertebrae	C 4
	5. Cervical vertebrae	C 5
	6. Cervical vertebrae	C 6
	7. Cervical vertebrae	C 7
Thoracic spine (12 vertebrae)	1. Thoracic vertebrae	Th 1
	2. Thoracic vertebrae	Th 2
	3. Thoracic vertebrae	Th 3
	4. Thoracic vertebrae	Th 4
	5. Thoracic vertebrae	Th 5
	6. Thoracic vertebrae	Th 6
	7. Thoracic vertebrae	Th 7
	8. Thoracic vertebrae	Th 8
	9. Thoracic vertebrae	Th 9
	10. Thoracic vertebrae	Th 10
	11. Thoracic vertebrae	Th 11
	12. Thoracic vertebrae	Th 12
Lumbar spine (5 vertebrae)	1. Lumbar vertebrae	L 1
	2. Lumbar vertebrae	L 2
	3. Lumbar vertebrae	L 3
	4. Lumbar vertebrae	L 4
	5. Lumbar vertebrae	L 5
	Sacrum	S 1
	Coccyx	S 2

1. **Cervical spine:** Seven vertebrae create the cervical spine, which is also known as the neck. This section of the spine is concave towards the posterior side of the body and convex towards the anterior side of the body.

   - There are a few specific vertebrae whose function is important to know and understand.
     1. C1: The first cervical vertebrae is also known as the atlas. The joint between the occiput (skull) and C1 (the atlas) allows for nodding of the head.
     2. C2: The second cervical vertebrae is known as the axis. The axis has a protrusion off the top of it which sits inside the ring formed by C1 (the atlas). The joint between C1 and C2 allows for 50% of the rotation in the neck.
   - The spine can move in any combination of six motions: flexion (forward bending), extension (backwards bending), right rotation, left rotation, right sidebending, and left sidebending. All six motions are performed by the cervical spine.

2. **Thoracic spine:** The thoracic spine consists of twelve vertebrae in the mid back. As a whole, this section of the spine is less mobile than both the cervical and lumbar spine. A large reason for this is the attachment of the ribcage. Despite the decreased mobility, the thoracic spine moves in all six of the same directions as the cervical spine. The curvature of the thoracic spine is opposite that of the cervical spine. It is concave towards the anterior side of the body and convex towards the posterior side of the body.

3. **Lumbar spine:** The lumbar spine is also known as the low back. It consists of the five vertebrae below the thoracic spine and above the sacrum. The body of the lumbar vertebrae are significantly larger than that of the cervical or thoracic vertebrae. This is due to the increased weight bearing needs of the low back. The lumbar spine moves in the same six directions as the rest of the spine. It has more range of motion than the thoracic spine but less than the cervical. The majority of rotation in the lumbar spine happens between L5 (the lowest lumbar vertebrae) and the sacrum. The curvature of the lumbar spine is in the same direction as the cervical spine, creating an S shaped curve throughout the spine as a whole.

- **Pelvis:**

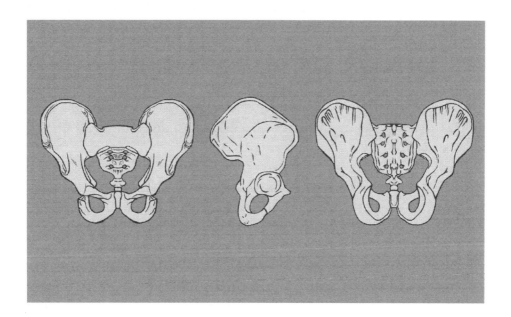

- The pelvis is a bowl shaped set of bones that consists of two pelvic bones (the left and right) as well as the sacrum. Each pelvic bone is comprised of three parts: the ilium (the pelvic crest), the ischium (the sitting bones), and the pubis (where the front of the pelvis connects). There is a joint between the pelvic bones at the pubis, where the left and right side meet at the anterior portion of the pelvis known as the pubic symphisis. At the posterior aspect of each pelvic bone and the sacrum the connection of these two bones forms the left and right sacroiliac (SI) joints. A small amount of movement occurs at each sacroiliac joint and this joint has many sensitive nerve endings. As a whole, the pelvis rotates both forward (anteriorly) and backwards (posteriorly). We discuss pelvic movement in depth below. The lateral portion of the pelvis forms the socket for the hip joint. The socket of the hip has significant depth and is much larger than the femoral head (ball) of the joint. This provides bony stability in the hip.

    - **Sacrum:**
        - The movement of the sacrum tilts both forward and backwards and is very closely related to the movement of the low back. As the low back flexes (rounds forward) the sacrum tilts posteriorly. As the low back extends (arches backwards) the sacrum tilts anteriorly. These motions also correspond to pelvic movement as a whole.
    - **Coccyx:**
        - The coccyx is a small triangular shaped bone that sits below the sacrum. It is commonly known as the tailbone.
    - **Pelvic movement:**

- Anterior pelvic tilt: The base (flat top) of the sacrum moves up and forward, pelvic bowl tilts forward (imagine that water would spill out the front if the pelvis was a bowl). This movement is associated with the lumbar spine finding extension (arching) such as during a backbend.
- Posterior pelvic tilt: The base of sacrum moves down and back, the pelvic bowl tilts backward (water would spill out the back), the pubic bone moves up and forward. During this movement the lumbar spine typically finds flexion (reversal of arch) such as during a forward fold.
- We typically want a "neutral pelvis" in yoga postures. For most people, this means a slight posterior tilt to remove the excess arch in the low back, but this may not be true for all. Some people naturally sit in a posterior pelvic tilt and require a small amount of anterior tilt to find neutral. It is important to avoid using broad cuing like "tuck the tailbone", as that can easily cause an over tilting posteriorly of the pelvis, completely reversing normal lumbar extension. Instead teach pelvic positions to your students and teach what a neutral pelvis and neutral lumbar spine feel like. Cat/cow and tabletop are excellent postures to use to teach these pelvic and lumbar positions.

- **Ribcage:**

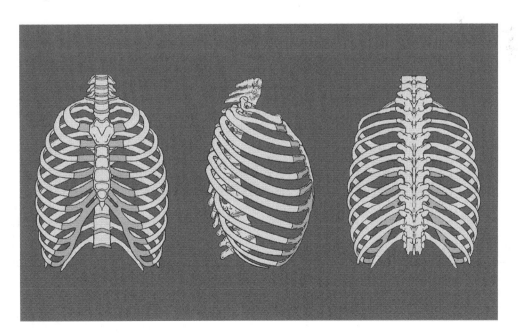

- The ribcage consists of twelve pairs of ribs that attach posteriorly to the thoracic spine and anteriorly to the sternum. The purpose of the ribcage is primarily to protect the heart and lungs. It also provides attachment points for musculature that is used to facilitate breathing.

- True ribs: Ribs one through seven are often referred to as "true ribs" as they each attach directly to the sternum.
- False ribs: Ribs eight through ten are often referred to as "false ribs" as they share a cartilage attachment to the sternum.
- Floating ribs: Ribs eleven and twelve are known as "floating ribs" as they do not attach to sternum at all..
- Sternum: The sternum is the bony breastplate at the anterior aspect of the chest.
- We often want students to open or broaden across their chest, the front side of their body, and their heart space. However, you must be careful of the language you use to cue this movement. Using cuing such as "open the heart towards the ceiling" can often cause over extension of the thoracic spine and protrusion of the lower ribcage. This disengages the abdominal muscles and puts the back at risk of injury. Use counter cues such as "tuck the front ribs" or "bring the front ribs and front of the pelvis closer together" to maintain length in the thoracic spine as the chest expands.

- **Upper extremity:**

  - **Clavicle:** The clavicle is also known as the collarbone. It's purpose is to act as a lever to facilitate elevation of the arm away from the torso. The distal (outer) end of the clavicle also helps to create the socket in which the ball of the humerus resides (forming the shoulder joint).
  - **Scapula:** The scapula is the triangular shaped bone that lies on the back side of the ribcage, also known as the shoulder blade. It attaches to the clavicle to complete the shoulder socket.
  - **Humerus:** The humerus is the upper arm bone. At the proximal (upper) end of the humerus is the head of the humerus, or the "ball" in the ball and socket joint that is the shoulder. This joint can move in many different directions: flexion, extension, abduction, adduction, internal rotation, and external rotation. The ball is significantly larger than the socket and therefore lacks bony stability. It's range of motion is significantly improved because of this lack of stability and it relies on muscular stability (from the rotator cuff, as mentioned previously) to keep proper alignment.
  - **Radius/Ulna:** These are the bones of the forearm. Where they meet the humerus forms the elbow joint. The elbow is a hinge joint and provides both flexion and extension (bending and straightening). The two bones of the forearm rotate upon each other allowing the palm of the hand to be flipped both up and down (called supination and pronation).

- **Carpals:** Eight carpal bones create the wrist joint. Because of the small nature of the carpal bones, the wrist is susceptible to injury by excessive force or prolonged time on the hands. Wrist pain and injuries are common in yoga.
- **Metacarpals:** These are the bones of the hand.
- **Phalanges:** These are the fingers.

- **Lower extremity:**

    - **Femur:** The femur is the long bone of the upper leg/thigh. The femoral head fits into the socket of the pelvis to create the hip joint. The hip joint is a ball and socket joint like and has all of the same motions as the shoulder. The hip joint, however, is much more stable than the shoulder due to its bony configuration. This means that the hip joint often needs mobility work (in yoga we call these postures "hip openers").
    - **Tibia/Fibula:** These are the bones of the lower leg. Where they meet the femur is known as the knee joint. This joint is similar to the elbow in that it is primarily a hinge joint, allowing bending and straightening.
    - **Tarsals:** Seven small bones make up the ankle. The ankle is very stable, especially in comparison to the wrist and has much lower incidence of injury in yoga.
    - **Metatarsals:** These are the foot bones. Their main purpose is to create the longitudinal arch in the foot which helps with stability in weightbearing.
    - **Phalanges:** Just like in the hand, the phalanges are the toes.

- **Skull:** While we typically view the skull as being one bone, it is actually a fusion of 22 smaller bones to create a protective covering for the brain.

Let's review of types of joints and joint mechanics:

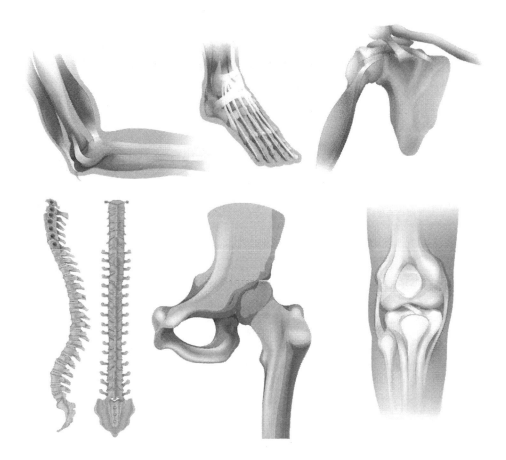

- **Ball and socket:** Both the hip and shoulder joints are ball and socket joints. They provide the greatest variety of motion (flexion, extension, abduction, adduction, internal rotation, external rotation). The hip has a deeper socket providing more bony stability but less mobility. The shoulder has a more shallow socket which results in a greater range of motion but more reliance on muscles, tendons, and ligaments for stability. Shoulder injuries are more common than hip injuries in yoga, as we'll see later.
- **Hinge:** Both the knee and elbow are hinge joints. These joints move primarily in flexion and extension (the knee does have a slight rotational component). This means that forcing rotation or torsion through these joints can cause injury.

To fully understand the different motions of these joints you must understand planes of movement.

- **Frontal:** The frontal plane is where abduction and adduction occur. Abduction is the motion of moving the arm or leg laterally away from the body. Adduction is the opposite motion, bringing the appendage back into the torso.
- **Sagittal:** The sagittal plane is where flexion and extension occur. Flexion is moving the arm overhead or the leg into the chest. Extension is lowering the arm or bringing the arm behind the torso as well as lowering the leg and bringing the leg behind the body. Flexion of the spine is folding forward and extension of the spine is moving to upright or arching backwards.
- **Transverse:** The transverse plane holds internal and external rotation, which primarily occur at the hip and shoulder. It is also where axial rotation (left and right rotation) of the spine occurs.

Understanding the anatomy and function of the major joints that make up the skeletal system is important for understanding how and why injury can occur. It also gives understanding to proper and improper alignment in yoga postures.

Nervous System:

To understand the nervous system is to understand the communication center of the body. The brain, the connection of the brain to the nerves, and the connection of the nerves to and from the body are what controls most bodily function.

Human Nervous System (Male & Female)

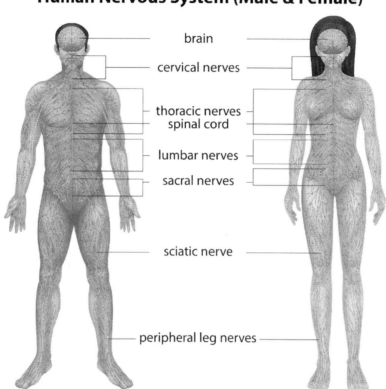

- **The Brain:** The control center of the body. As a yoga instructor, it is less important to know the specific names and locations of the different areas of the brain as it is to understand how they function. Each section of the brain is responsible for something different. There's an auditory section (hearing), a visual section (sight), an olfactory section (smell), etc. Previously it was thought that once the brain matured in young adulthood, it didn't have the capacity to change. We now know that is false. The brain can create new pathways and connections in response to stimulus given to the body. In a sense, it can be re-wired. This means changes in behaviors, patterns, thoughts, and activity can alter the brain (both positively and negatively). There has been extensive research done on the effects of yoga and meditation on the brain connections, pathways, and activation which supports this theory of elasticity and the brain's ability to change.

- **The Spinal Cord:** You can think of the spinal cord as the information superhighway. It connects the brain to the external world, taking signals both from the brain to the body and vice versa. And it does this very quickly. Research has shown that these nerve impulses travel at an average speed of around 100 meters/second (about 350 feet/second). Much of this transmission happens below your conscious awareness.

- **Spinal Nerves:** Spinal nerves exit from levels of the spinal cord to innervate different areas of the body. They can be separated into two types of nerves: afferent (nerves that bring information from the external world to the body) and efferent (nerves that bring action from the brain to the body). Afferent nerves are also known as sensory nerves and efferent nerves are also known as motor nerves. We will discuss these more deeply below.

  - **Motor nerves:** When the brain (consciously or subconsciously) decides to cause an action to happen, that signal gets transmitted from the brain to the spinal cord to muscles to cause that action via motor (efferent) nerves.
  - **Sensory nerves:** When the body experiences something (a smell, touch, heat, sound, sight, etc.) from the external world, that information gets sent from to the brain via sensory (afferent) nerves and the spinal cord.

- **Autonomic Nervous System:** The autonomic nervous system is the part of the nervous system that is responsible for many of the bodily functions that are not consciously controlled. For example, the heart rate, the blood pressure, and digestion. It is split into two sections - the sympathetic nervous system and the parasympathetic nervous system. However, try not to view these sections as one OR the other, instead think of the ANS as a sliding scale. At any given point your body is functioning somewhere along the spectrum between the sympathetic nervous system and the parasympathetic nervous system, and it's fluctuating constantly. Also try to avoid labelling one as "good" and the other as "bad". Both have their appropriate times and purposes for functioning.

  - **Sympathetic Nervous System:** This nervous system is sometimes called the "fight or flight" system. When it is overactive, one might experience elevated heart rate, elevated respiratory rate, elevated blood pressure, decreased digestion, and the feelings of anxiety or stress. Due to the overstimulating nature of our current society, many people live in a state of overactive SNS. Their body is reacting as though it is in physical danger and must be ready to fight or run, even though the physical threat does not exist. The body continues to perceive emotional or mental threats the same as it once (evolutionarily) perceived a physical threat. Most of the nerves of the SNS exit from thoracic spine region.

  - **Parasympathetic Nervous System:** This is sometimes known as the "rest and digest" nervous system. When one's body feels safe and properly cared for, it is existing in a primarily parasympathetic state. The heart rate and blood pressure are lower, the digestive system is getting optimal blood flow, and the higher cortical (emotional, memory, and processing) parts of the brain can be active. The body does not perceive threat so it feels like it can distribute its resources to other, restorative functions. Yoga, meditation, and pranayama work can all help people move more towards this end of the spectrum. Most of the PNS nerves exit from the cranium/cervical spine and sacral regions.

- It's important to remember that both ends of the autonomic nervous system spectrum hold value. Yoga can help with educating people on how to move along the spectrum as well as facilitating techniques that can cause a shift and change.

Cardiovascular System:

The main function of the cardiovascular system is to pump blood throughout the body. Metrics (ways to measure the efficiency and health of the cardiovascular system) include blood pressure and heart rate.

Blood Flow of the Human Heart

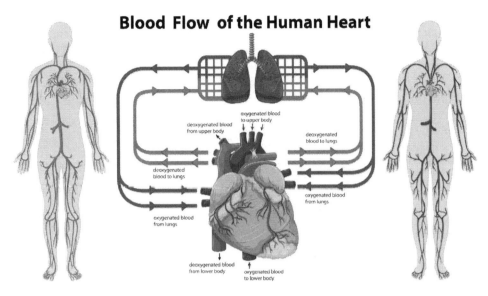

- **Heart**: The heart is a muscle that lies just to the left of center in the chest cavity. The heart's primary function is the movement of blood (and therefore oxygen) throughout the body. It does this through a series of contractions which creates a pumping mechanism. The heart is separated into two sides (the left and right) and each side is separated into halves (the upper half is referred to as the atrium and the lower half is the ventricle). The left side of the heart pumps oxygenated blood to the rest of the body while the right side of the heart pumps deoxygenated blood back to the lungs. The rate at which the heart pumps is measured as the heart rate (in beats per minute).
- The flow of blood in the body and through the heart is as follows:
    - Oxygen enters the lungs through an inhale and gets exchanged with outgoing carbon dioxide to oxygenate the blood.
    - This oxygenated blood flows via the pulmonary veins into the left atrium.
    - From the left atrium it moves to the left ventricle.
    - It gets pumped out of the left ventricle via the aorta and travels to the rest of the body to oxygenate cells.
    - When this is complete, the deoxygenated blood heads back to the heart via the superior and inferior vena cava and into the right atrium.
    - It flows from the right atrium to the right ventricle.
    - It gets pumped from the right ventricle back to the lungs to begin the process again.

- Arteries always take blood away from the heart and veins always take blood towards the heart.

Respiratory System:

The respiratory system is the system of breathing. The purpose of breathing is to take in oxygen to fuel the cells of the body and to expel carbon dioxide, a waste product of our body. Breathing is one of only two bodily functions that happen both consciously and subconsciously. The other is blinking. This means we breathe automatically, but that we can also control and regulate our breathing.

Anatomy of Human Lungs

larynx

trachea (windpipe)

right superior lobe

left superior lobe

bronchial tree

bronchi

right middle lobe

pleura

right inferior lobe

left inferior lobe

diaphragm

- **Lungs**: The lungs are the organs of breathing. They are well protected within the ribcage and consist of elastic sacs (you can envision them as being similar to a balloon) with branching passageways into which air is drawn. The lungs sit atop the diaphragm, which is the main muscle of respiration. The diaphragm is a double domed muscle that separates the abdominal cavity (where your abdominal organs exist) and the thoracic cavity (where your heart and lungs reside). When you inhale, the diaphragm contracts and moves downward, therefore creating more space in the thoracic cavity, which lowers the pressure relative to outside of the body. This causes the inhalation. When you exhale, the diaphragm relaxes and returns to its upward resting position, facilitating removal of air from the lungs. A diagram to illustrate breathing is noted below.

- The amount of air we can hold in our lungs is known as our lung capacity. During normal, resting, everyday breathing we typically use a small portion of our total maximum lung capacity. Introducing breathing exercises (pranayama) can help improve lung function and capacity.

- Mechanics of breathing:

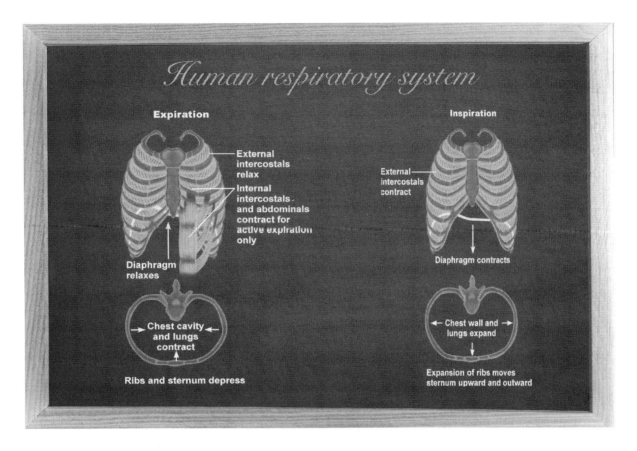

Digestive System:

Digestion is the process that occurs from the moment that food or liquid enters the body through the mouth until the moment that it leaves the body through excretion. The digestive system is the system of organs that allows digestion to take place. While the digestive system is complex and important, the details aren't necessary for yoga instructors. We will go over how the nervous system affects the digestive system as well as which poses are helpful for the digestive system. Teachers and students are encouraged to engage in more specific research if digestion is something that interests them.

Human Digestive System

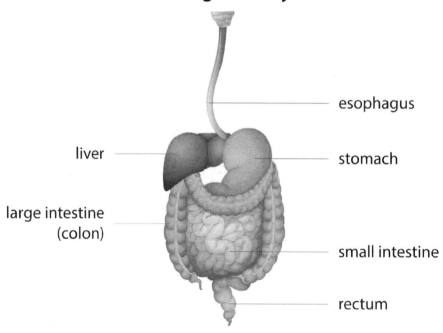

esophagus

liver

stomach

large intestine
(colon)

small intestine

rectum

- **Nervous system control:**
    - While the sympathetic nervous system is engaged and the body is in "fight or flight" mode, the majority of the blood stays in the extremities (muscles of the arms and/or legs) and out of the digestive system. Digestion is not an immediate need when the sympathetic system is engaged. Therefore, ingested food tends to pause in the digestive system without the body absorbing the nutrients until the body begins to move towards the parasympathetic end of the spectrum. The body doesn't always go immediately back to normal. Sometimes the digestive system is sped up, which can result in problems like diarrhea.

- Chronic stress and activation of the sympathetic nervous system causes confusion and chaos in the digestive system and can cause chronic digestive illness, problems with absorbing nutrients, and dysfunction digesting food.
- Yoga and meditation principles can encourage people to be more on the parasympathetic or "rest and digest" side of the spectrum, which results in increased blood flow to the digestive organs, normal hormonal regulation of digestion, and therefore better digestion.

- **Yoga Postures:**
  - Twists are great postures for digestion and cleansing. Think of twisting as acting similarly to wringing out a sponge. When you twist, you squeeze abdominal organs which facilitates flow of the digestive juices and contents of the digestive system, as well as temporarily cutting off blood supply to that organ. When the twist is released, flow of new blood flushes into the organ. You should always encourage twisting to the right before twisting to the left for improvement in digestive function, as this facilitates the normal flow of digestion in a clockwise pattern through the intestines. Malasana (yogi squat) is also an excellent posture for digestion. The squatting position places the lower intestines into a more ergonomically correct position to help speed up elimination.

Endocrine System:

Your endocrine system is the regulatory system of your body. It consists of glands that release hormones, as well as the hormones they release. Hormones can be thought of as the keys to your body. When they interact with the correct receptors they cause certain things to either start or stop happening. Similar to the digestive system, we will discuss how yoga can impact the endocrine system. The endocrine system is very complex and education can go far beyond what is included here. If students or teachers are interested in the endocrine system, they are encouraged to study on their own.

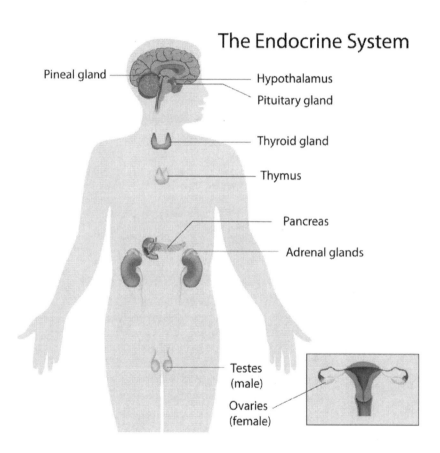

The Endocrine System

Pineal gland

Hypothalamus

Pituitary gland

Thyroid gland

Thymus

Pancreas

Adrenal glands

Testes
(male)

Ovaries
(female)

- **Glands of the Endocrine System:**
    - **Pituitary gland**: The pituitary gland is located in the base of the brain and is often referred to as the "master gland". It is responsible for releasing hormones that help control growth, blood pressure, the thyroid gland, and metabolism. It also plays a function in temperature regulation and pain relief. Essentially, the pituitary gland impacts the function of many other areas of the endocrine system. Inversions are the group of postures that help stimulate this gland. They include:

forearm stand, headstand, handstand, and wheel (to name a few). Increasing the blood flow to the brain through these inversions helps stimulate pituitary function.
- **Thyroid and parathyroid glands**: The thyroid and parathyroid glands are located in the anterior region of the neck. Thyroid function controls your basal metabolic rate (base metabolism) and functional metabolism. The parathyroid helps control the amount of different minerals in the body. Postures that promote increased blood flow and stimulation of these glands include eagle arms, bridge, cow face pose, and shoulderstand. The action of drawing the chin in towards the chest (jalandhara bandha) in these poses is the action which stimulates these glands.
- **Adrenal glands**: The adrenal glands are just above the kidneys, on the left and right sides of the low back. They are responsible for secretion of adrenaline and cortisol. The hormone adrenaline is responsible for increasing heart rate, blood pressure, and preparing the body for a "fight or flight" response in a stressful situation. Cortisol functions to raise the blood sugar and prepare the muscles for the same reaction (giving the muscles the fuel they will need in a fight or flight situation). Long term, high levels of cortisol can have a immunosuppressive effect (weakening the immune system). Overactivity of the adrenal glands due to chronic stress can result in what's known as "adrenal fatigue", where the body becomes depleted and exhausted. Poses such as a supported seated forward fold, legs up the wall, supported bridge, and savasana done in a restorative setting can help combat this fatigue.
- **Pancreas**: The pancreas is located behind the stomach and is responsible for secreting insulin (which regulates blood sugar levels) as well as many digestive enzymes (which assist in breakdown of carbohydrates, proteins, and fats). The pancreas can be stimulated by seated spinal twists, plough pose, seated forward fold, and peacock.
- **Reproductive organs (ovaries/testicles)**: These male and female sex organs control androgens (male sex hormones like testosterone) and estrogen (female sex hormones). Many poses can help stimulate these organs to regulate and improve the release of the sex hormones. These poses include double pigeon, cobbler's pose, and legs up the wall.

important to know the structural anatomy of the body, it's more pertinent for the yoga r to understand how that anatomy applies to the body during a yoga practice.

ɪ... ɪlowing section of this handbook reviews some of the most common yoga injuries, what causes them, how they can be prevented, and modifications that can be offered to students.

It is important to remember that as a yoga instructor, you are not a doctor or physical therapist. You can not diagnose or treat pain or injuries. It's always best to refer students out to see a doctor or therapist if they tell you they are experiencing pain or some injury.

Common Yoga Injuries:

While injuries in yoga are less common than in other high impact or contact sports, they do occur. Poor alignment in postures or overuse of specific body structures will lead to chronic injuries. Traumatic injuries occur less frequently. In this course we will examine the most common yoga injuries and causes, joint by joint.

Cervical Spine (Neck):
- Most common injuries: Muscle strains and nerve impingement.
- Causes:
    - Over rotation of the neck during postures like side angle lunge or triangle. When the neck rotates without being in perfect alignment, pressure can be placed on the joints between the vertebrae.
    - Hyperextension (or dropping back of the head) in postures like upward facing dog or camel will also put undue pressure on the back of the neck, specifically at the C1/C2 level just below the skull. Not only is this dangerous for the spine, but also can compromise blood flow to the brain.
    - Poor alignment in shoulderstand or headstand can place excess weight and stress on the structures of the neck.
- Prevention:
    - Instruct students to turn their head and look up in postures only if it feels good to them. Remind them to keep a neutral and long neck.
    - Properly instruct poses such as shoulderstand and headstand and ensure students have proper alignment once in those postures.
- Modifications:
    - The neck can always stay in neutral, eyes facing the same direction as shoulders, in order to prevent rotational injury.
    - Replacement of the inversions listed above with legs up the wall is an excellent modification for students with neck pain or injury.

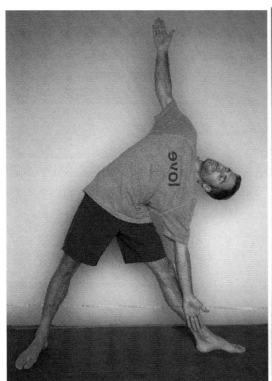 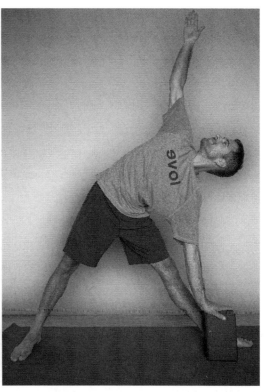

Triangle - Poor Cervical Alignment   Triangle - Correct Cervical Alignment

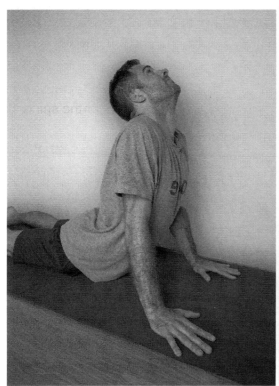 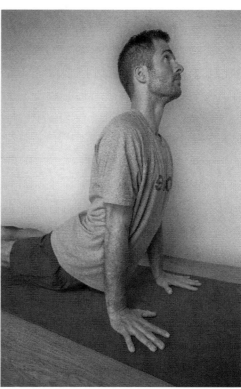

Upward Facing Dog - Poor Cervical Alignment   Upward Facing Dog - Correct Cervical Alignment

Shoulder:
- Most Common Injuries: Pinching or partial tears of the rotator cuff.
- Causes:
    - Because these are small muscles, they are overworked easily. Vinyasa style classes with many chaturangas are a cause of injury, especially due to typically poor alignment during chaturanga.
    - Another common cause of injury is forcing binds in different postures. Binding requires a large range of internal rotation in the shoulder joint and forcing binds (or being adjusted to go deeper into a bind) can easily cause injury.
- Prevention:
    - Take the time to properly teach chaturanga, as well as modifications if chaturanga cannot be performed properly.
    - Encourage external rotation of the shoulders in postures that have extended arms. Instruct students to rotate the pinkies in and the thumbs out. This position seats the ball of the shoulder joint firmly into the socket, which protects it and strengthens the stabilizing muscles.
    - Cue students into and out of binds slowly and with care. Reinforce the importance of an open chest and retracted scapulae.
- Modifications:
    - Chaturangas can be performed on the knees or not at all, moving straight from plank to downward facing dog.
    - Students with shoulder pain can extend their arms straight in front of them instead of overhead.
    - Binds can be performed with a strap to ensure proper alignment.

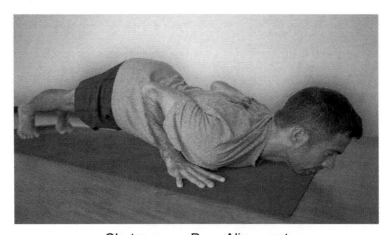

Chaturanga - Poor Alignment

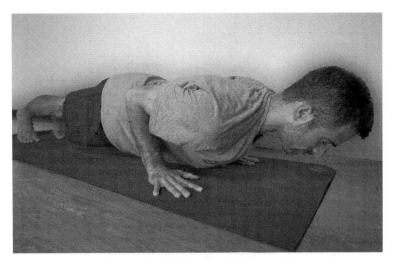

Chaturanga - Correct Alignment

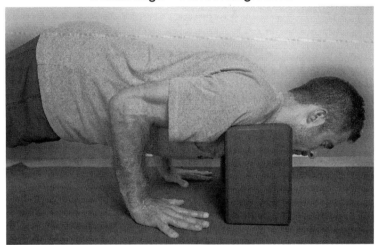

Chaturanga - Correct Alignment with Blocks

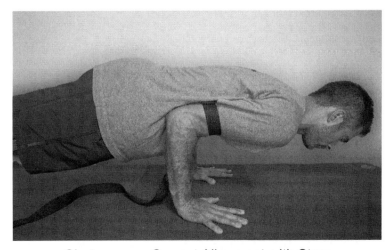

Chaturanga - Correct Alignment with Strap

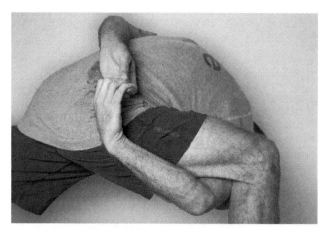

Bind - Incorrect, Posterior View

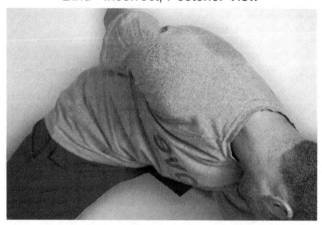

Bind - Incorrect, Anterior View

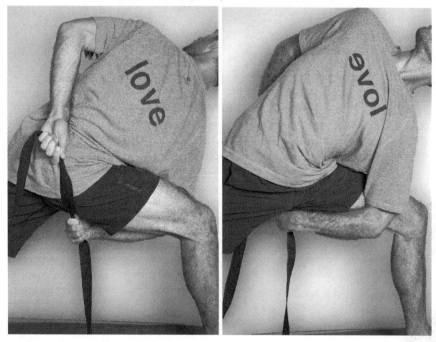

Bind - Correct, Posterior View   Bind - Correct, Anterior View

Wrist:

- Most Common Injuries: Overuse injury of the ligaments or tendons that support the small bones of the wrist.
- Causes:
    - Because we don't often spend time on our hands outside of the yoga studio, the repetition of weight being placed through the hands on the floor in different postures causes strain or sprain of the tendons or ligaments of the wrist and hand.
    - Poor understanding of hasta bandha (the hand lock, hand position on the floor) can also lead to improper forces through the wrist.
- Prevention:
    - Teach hasta bandha to all students. Remind them throughout class to find proper hand alignment when hands are in contact with the floor.
    - Include active wrist stretches during the yoga class.
- Modifications:
    - Students can use forearms on the mat for poses like plank (forearm plank), up dog (sphinx), and downward facing dog (dolphin).
    - Students can also rest on the knuckles, making a fist, to ensure good alignment of the wrist.

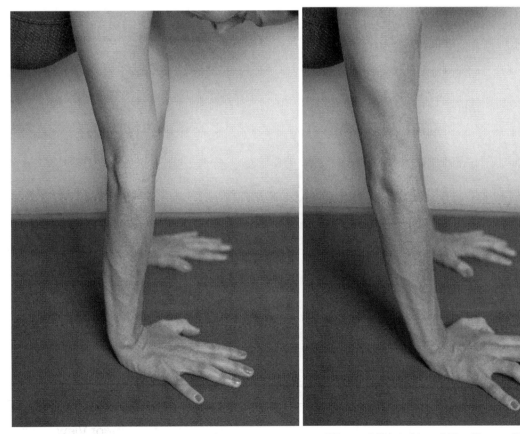

Elbow, Wrist, Hand Position - Incorrect   Elbow, Wrist, Hand Position - Correct

Lumbar Spine (Low Back):

- Most Common Injuries: Nerve impingement, muscle strain, or disc injury.
- Causes:
  - Improper mechanics in large range of motion postures like forward folds and backbends.
- Prevention:
  - Proper warm up of the spine and its associated musculature. For backbends, this means proper opening of the hip flexors and latissimus and proper activation of the core.
  - In forward folds, it is important to keep a neutral lumbar spine, especially if the posture includes any element of rotation.
  - In backbends, it is essential to keep engagement of the core to protect the lumbar spine as well as to create length in the hip flexors to allow the pelvis and hip to move in conjunction with the spine. You should also be aware of any instances of hinging at the low back versus a smooth backbend.
- Modification:
  - Encourage bending the knees in a forward fold to protect the low back from injury.
  - Modifying deep backbends by replacing them with more moderate backbends is smart for students with low back pain. For example, bridge instead of wheel or cobra instead of upward facing dog.

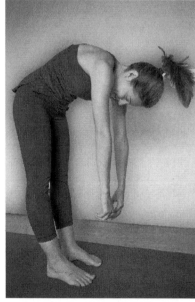 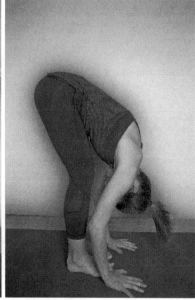 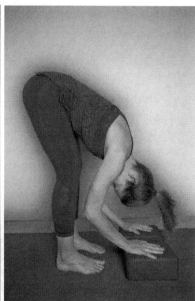

Forward Fold - Incorrect   Forward Fold - Correct   Forward Fold - Correct, Blocks

Knee:

- Most Common Injuries: Remember that the knee is a primary hinge joint, with just a small amount of rotation. Knee injuries can occur if too much rotation is introduced (such as transitioning from an open hip to a closed hip posture) or if the knee is hyperextended.
- Causes:
  - Transitions such as warrior 2 to warrior 1 and reverse warrior to low lunge can cause torsion or twisting through the knee.
  - Forcing the legs into lotus (or half lotus) without having proper hip mobility.
  - Hyperextension of the knee in postures such as triangle or skandasana.
- Prevention:
  - Cue students to activate their quadriceps and find a microbend in the extended knee during all straight legged postures to avoid hyperextension of the knee.
  - Properly increase rotation of the hips before introducing postures such as lotus, half lotus, or even pigeon.
- Modifications:
  - Using blocks to maintain hip alignment in postures such as half or full pigeon is excellent.

General Techniques to Prevent Yoga Injury:

- First and foremost, you must understand anatomy and biomechanics! Having this solid foundation with help you to be able to safely sequence a class, properly warm students up for more challenging postures, be able to accurately cue alignment in different poses, and be able to correctly adjust students.

- Clearly instruct students to listen to their own body. Each body is different and each pose will feel different to each person. Students should be reminded to ease into and out of poses and to only take postures if they feel good. Students should always feel welcome to modify or skip postures all together.

- Properly sequence classes for warm up, muscle and joint preparation, and safety.
  - Proper sequencing for backbends includes:
    - Activation of the anterior core musculature.
    - Lengthening and stretching of the hip flexors, latissimus, and triceps.
    - Pay mind to open the hips and shoulders with smaller amplitude backbends before going for a peak pose.
  - Proper sequencing for inversions includes:
    - Activation of all four sides of the core, the glutes, the quadriceps, and the latissimus to ensure proper co-contraction of these muscles for stability in the inversion.
    - Opening and stretching the latissimus, especially for handstand and forearm stand.

- Ensure that the neck has been safely warmed up prior to attempting any weight bearing inversion such as a headstand.
    - Proper sequencing for forward folds includes:
        - Activation of the quadriceps to help protect the hamstrings while in a forward fold.
        - Gentle lengthening and opening of low back musculature and hamstrings prior to a deep forward bend.
        - Ensure that the spine has been warmed up in all six directions of movement.
    - Proper sequencing for arm balances includes:
        - Preparation of shoulder girdle stabilizers (rotator cuff), forearm musculature, and core strength.
        - Warming up and preparing the joints of the wrist as well as the shoulder will help students be ready for an arm balance.

- Intently observe your students during class. Verbally or physically assist to correct students in postures that may cause injury. Try to move around the room so that you can see all of the students from many angles while teaching.

- Take care with adjustments. Have an intention, be firm, sync with the student's breath, notice if the student seems uncomfortable. Only adjust students that you are comfortable with, in poses that you are comfortable adjusting.

When a student has pain or is injured:
- Do not try to diagnose the problem. Know who to refer the student to, whether it's a physical therapist, chiropractor, or doctor, have people in the community you know and trust. It is outside of your scope of practice to diagnose or give specific advice regarding injuries.

- Know the difference between pain and discomfort and what questions to ask to determine which the student is experiencing. Many people don't know the difference. Sharp, shooting, radiating, burning are all words that describe pain. Achy and dull indicate more of a discomfort feeling. Remind students that their experience of pain is going to be unique to them and that they should always listen to and trust their body.

- Always encourage students not to push through pain (or significant discomfort) and to rest/avoid postures as needed. Each person's body is different, therefore poses are going to feel different on different people.

Definitions and Concepts in Practical Anatomy

Understanding the concepts and language used in talking about the body with regards to yoga is important for properly instructing and conveying concepts. Below we define and discuss some of this language.

Stretching or Lengthening Muscles:
- To stretch or lengthen a muscle is to move the two attachment points away from each other, causing the muscle to get longer. Static stretches are held for a prolonged period of time, and most yoga postures are static holds.

- Different ways to stretch a muscle, safely and effectively include:
    - "Stretch an active muscle": Maintaining a degree of engagement in the muscle group being stretched will prevent it from being overstretched or damaged. For example, if you are stretching the hamstring in a seated forward fold, you should maintain a slight activation of the hamstring throughout the posture in order to protect the hamstring from over stretching.
    - Reciprocal Inhibition: Reciprocal inhibition is the process of muscles on one side of a joint relaxing to accommodate contraction on the other side of that joint. To use the hamstring stretch example, gently contracting the quadriceps (the muscle group opposite the hamstring) with cause a deeper relaxation and therefore ability to lengthen the hamstrings.

Strengthening muscles:
- There are three types of contractions that cause strengthening of muscles.
    - Concentric contractions: Cause the muscle to shorten and change the angle of the joint. These are good for moving an external load (or body weight). An example is to look at the quadriceps during utkatasana (chair pose). When returning to standing from chair, the quadriceps shorten resulting in a concentric contraction.
    - Eccentric contractions: Cause the muscle to decelerate a movement or otherwise control the repositioning of a load, causing a lengthening of the muscle. This is essential for controlling movement and transitions. Using the chair pose example, the quadriceps undergo an eccentric contraction when lowering to chair from standing.
    - Isometric contractions: The joint angle and muscle length do not change. Good for creating and maintaining stability and balance. While holding chair, the quadriceps experience an isometric contraction. Once in a posture, most muscles are contracting isometrically to hold that posture.

Joint mechanics:
- Certain patterns in different joints work together the best to result in the most motion with the least restriction. In yoga, the most important of these occur in the spine.

- Cervical spine: When side bending (lateral flexion), rotation to the same side occurs. Think of this when asking students to look in certain directions in poses. For example, in triangle pose, if you want a student to look up towards their top hand, they must side bend the neck slightly in that same direction. Gravity will have the tendency to side bend the neck the opposite direction so the student must fight gravity.

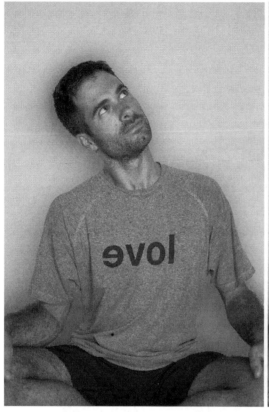 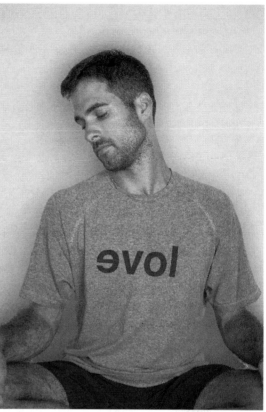

Cervical Rotation - Incorrect   Cervical Rotation - Correct

- Lumbar spine: When sidebending (lateral flexion), rotation to the opposite side occurs. Think of this when performing postures like utthita parsvakonasana.

- Capsular/closed packed position: The joint has the least space and is most at risk for injury.
    - Shoulder: Full abduction and internal rotation. This is why in most yoga postures we encourage external rotation of the shoulders to maintain space and safety.

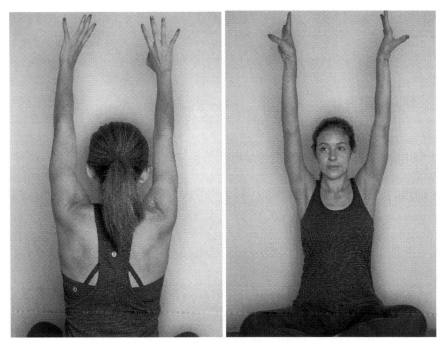

Overhead Reaching - Internal Rotation, Incorrect

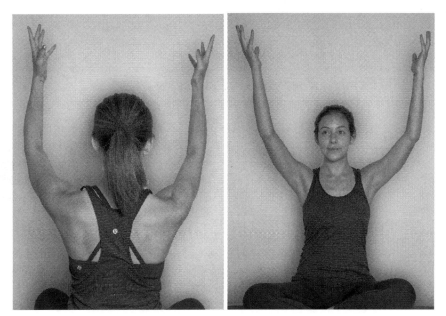

Overhead Reaching - External Rotation, Correct

Review of Groups of Yoga Postures:
This review will discuss each group of postures, which muscles are most involved, which joints are involved, important biomechanics to remember, and some example postures.

Standing Postures:
- General muscle groups involved: quadriceps, glutes, hamstrings, calves, foot/ankle muscles.
- Joints/alignment: ankles, knees, hips, spine.
- Important biomechanics: hip rotation positions (open hip versus closed hip).
- Example pose(s):
    - Warrior 1 (Virabhadrasana 1): This is a closed hip posture, which means both hips face forward.
        - It is important to look at alignment of front knee over front ankle facing over the second toe.
        - The back foot is at 45 degrees, with the outer edge of the foot pressing into the mat.
        - The inner arches of both feet are lifted.
        - The spine is in neutral, sitting bones pointing towards the ground, and the lower abdomen is engaged.
    - Warrior 2 (Virabhadrasana 2): This is an open hip posture, which means at least one of the hips is externally rotated.
        - Like in Warrior 1, the front knee should be stacked over the front ankle, with the foot over the second toe.
        - The back foot is at 90 degrees with weight pressed through the outer foot.
        - Again, both inner arches should be lifted.
        - The spine should be erect and stacked with the shoulders directly over the hips and the arms extended parallel to the floor at the level of the shoulders.

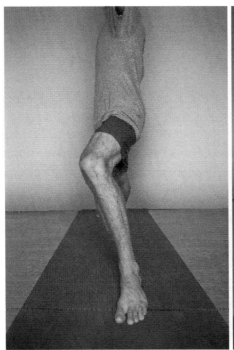

Warrior 2 - Incorrect Knee Alignment   Warrior 2 - Correct Knee Alignment

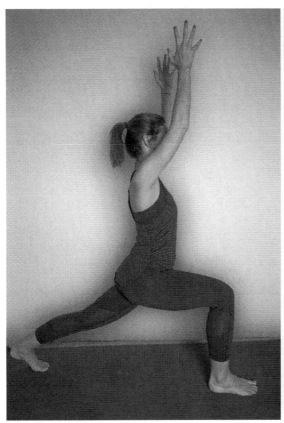
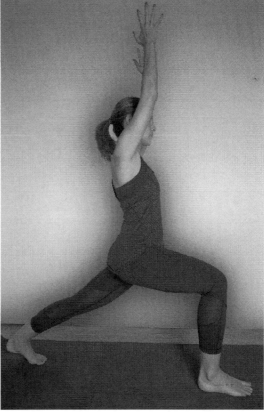

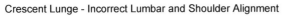
Crescent Lunge - Incorrect Lumbar and Shoulder Alignment   Crescent Lunge - Correct Lumbar and Shoulder Alignment

Balance Postures:

- General muscle groups involved: ankle/foot stabilizers, calves, glutes, hamstrings, quads, abdominals, obliques, back musculature.
- Joints/alignment: ankles, knees, hips, spine.
- Important biomechanics: upright postural alignment and common compensations for weak gluteus medius(uneven pelvis or leaning to one side).
- Example pose(s):
    - Tree (Vrksasana): In tree pose, the shoulders should stack over the hips and the hips over the standing ankle. It is important to activate the transverse abdominis in order to neutralize the lumbar spine and protect the low back.
    - Standing Hand to Big Toe (Uttitha Hasta Padangusthasana): This pose has similar alignment cues to tree pose. As the student reaches for the knee or big toe to begin to extend the leg, continue to reinforce upright posture, even hips, and erect spine.

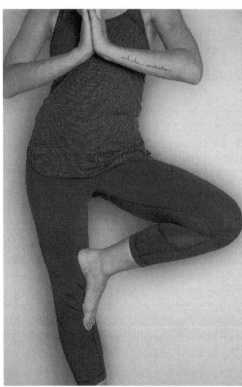
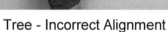
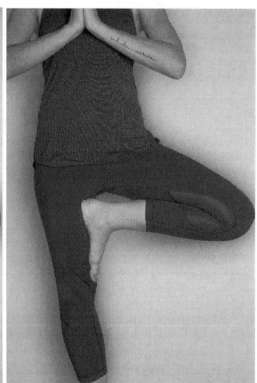

Tree - Incorrect Alignment   Tree - Correct Alignment

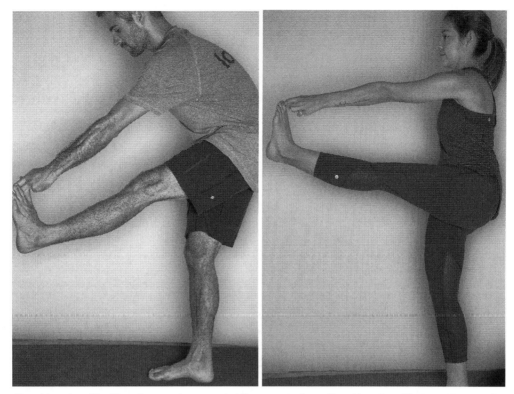

Standing Hand to Big Toe Pose - Incorrect Alignment Standing Hand to Big Toe Pose - Correct Alignment

Backbends:

- General muscle groups involved: back musculature, glutes, hamstrings, calves, periscapular muscles, latissimus dorsi, wrist/forearm stabilizers.
- Joints/alignment: knees, hips, spine, shoulders, elbows, wrists.
- Important biomechanics: shoulder mobility (postures to maximize shoulder flexion), hip flexor length, distribution of backbend throughout the spine versus a hinge point.
- Example pose(s):
    - Upward Facing Dog (Urdhva Mukha Svanasana): This is a large backbend that requires warm up prior to moving into.
        - The student should demonstrate activation of the quadriceps by pressing the tops of the feet into the ground and lifting the knees, minimal activation of the glutes to protect the low back, deep core (transversus) engagement to continue to elongate the spine in the backbend, and downward pressure of the hands in order to lift the head away from the shoulders and maintain length in the neck.
        - The student should also look forward (versus upward) to protect the cervical spine.
    - Wheel (Urdhva Dhanurasana): This is a large backbend which also incorporates a significant level of shoulder mobility.
        - In addition to many of the same cues as the previous backbend, students must be able to achieve full shoulder flexion in order to safely perform

wheel. This means opening of the triceps and latissimus prior to moving into the pose.
- This pose also requires significant hip extension and hip flexor mobility.
- The combination of open shoulders and hips along with core activation will allow this deep backbend to be equally distributed throughout the spine.

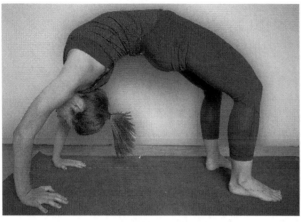 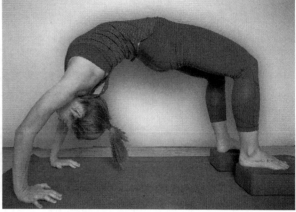

Wheel - Improper Alignment (hinge)   Wheel - Proper Alignment, with Blocks

Forward Bends:
- General muscle groups involved: anterior core, low back, hamstrings, calves, quadriceps.
- Joints/alignment: spine, hips, knees.
- Important biomechanics: understanding the position of lumbar spine and pelvis in forward bends, understanding the compensations that occur when hamstring length is compromised.
- Example pose(s):
  - Seated Forward Fold (Paschimottanasana): The objective is to maintain a neutral lumbar spine as the thoracic and cervical spine relax forward towards the lower part of the legs. For many people, this will mean coming into the forward fold (and possibly maintaining the forward fold) with knee flexion in order to keep the neutral lumbar spine. This is fine as a hamstring stretch will still be felt with the knees bent. Encouragement of length on the inhales and depth on the exhales is proper cuing for deepening the pose.
  - Standing Forward Fold (Uttanasana): The alignment and cuing for this posture is similar to that of a seated forward fold. However, because this pose is done against gravity, extra care must be maintained to keep a neutral lumbar spine. Over rounding of the spine against gravity can result in low back injury. Forcing of a deeper fold in this posture can also result in hamstring strain or injury. It may feel better for students to maintain feet at hips width apart to protect both the hamstrings and the low back.

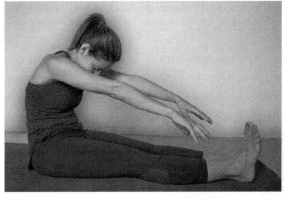
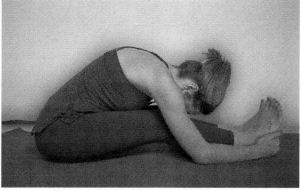

Seated Forward Fold - Incorrect Alignment   Seated Forward Fold - Correct Alignment

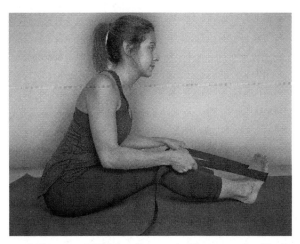

Seated Forward Fold - Correct Alignment with Strap

Twists:
- General muscle groups involved: low back, obliques, abdominals.
- Joints/alignment: spine, hips, shoulders.
- Important biomechanics: Understand the difference between closed twists and open twists (a closed twist is when the shoulders and hips rotate opposite directions and an open twist is when the rotate the same direction), be observant of cervical and lumbar spine positions (keep spine in neutral while twisting - avoid both flexion and extension during rotation).
- Example pose(s):
    - Seated Twist/Half Lord of the Fishes (Ardha Matseyendrasana): This posture is a closed twist (with the shoulders and hips rotating in opposite directions).
        - It is essential that each inhale results in extension and lengthening of the spine before rotating deeper with the exhale.
        - Ensure that the lumbar spine is in neutral. If you see it in flexion, the student can extend the bottom leg or sit on a block or prop.
        - Also be aware of the depth of cervical rotation and avoiding over rotating the neck.

- Extended Side Angle (Utthita Parsvakonasana): This is an open twist, with the shoulders and hips rotating the same direction (just to different depths). It is easy for the spine to sidebend in the direction of the earth due to gravity in this posture, so encourage the use of props to maintain length in both sides of the spine and encourage a neutral neck prior to rotating the head either direction.

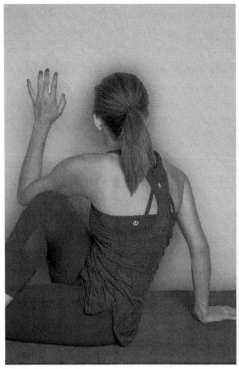 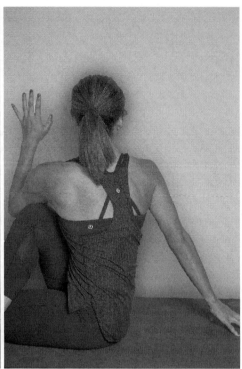

Spinal Twist- Improper Alignment   Spinal Twist- Proper Alignment

Inversions:
- General muscle groups involved: all.
- Joints/alignment: spine.
- Important biomechanics: spinal alignment (especially in headstand variations)..
- Example pose(s):
    - Headstand (Sirsasana): This is an excellent inversion, bringing blood flow to the brain, improving energy, and challenging the physical body. However, neck injuries are fairly common in headstand due to improper cervical spine alignment as well as inadequate strength and stability in the shoulders to support the weight of the body upside down. Education on location of the crown of the head is important as well as education on proper unweighting of the head through use of upper body strength.

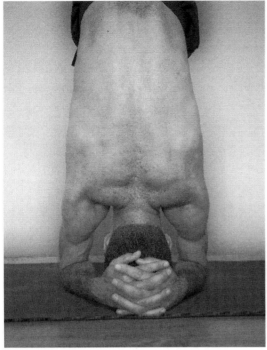 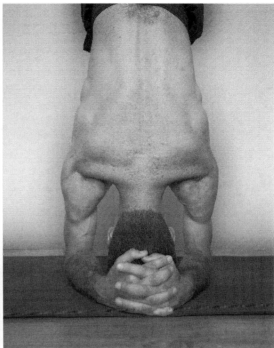

Headstand - Incorrect Alignment   Headstand - Correct Alignment

Arm Balances:
- General muscle groups: core, upper body.
- Joints/alignment: shoulders, elbows, wrists.
- Important biomechanics: proper upper extremity alignment (ability to find and maintain the same arm position as in chaturanga, keeping elbows in line with the shoulders and stacking the upper extremity joints), core stability and strength (ability to maintain engagement of the transverse abdominis to unweight and support the body).
- Example pose(s):
    - Crow (Bakasana): In crow pose, the upper body must be able to find similar alignment to chaturanga in order for the shoulders to maintain their stability and strength while holding the weight of the body.
        - Look for the elbows bowing to the outside as well as the shoulders dipping forward.
        - It's also important to maintain an active core to help support the weight of the body as opposed to the weight being dumped on just the arms.

Hip Openers:
- General muscle groups: hip flexors, hip rotators (internal and external), hip adductors.
- Joints/alignment: hips, knees, lumbar spine.
- Important biomechanics: understanding the motion and positions of the hips (remember that the hip moves in six directions, therefore "hip opening" is not just postures that externally rotate the hips), protecting distal joints (if the hips are not open enough in certain postures the knee can be compromised or rotated).

- Example poses:
    - Half Pigeon (Eka Pada Kapotasana): This is a typical "hip opening" posture, meaning it stretches and lengthens the internal rotators and extensors of the hip by placing the hip in external rotation and flexion. It is important to support the pelvis in whatever degree of rotation is available at the hip so that the knee does not become compromised. It is important to remember that all hips are anatomically different, so hip opening postures will look different on each person.
    - Hero's Pose (Virasana): This is essentially the opposite of half pigeon - it stretches the external rotators and the hip flexors (when in a reclined position). This is another posture where the knee can be easily compromised. The hips can be supported with a block and reclining should be avoided until the hips have adequate range of motion to support the knee.

It is important to remember that this book and the associated manual are intended to provide a base level of practical understanding of anatomy. This is just the introduction to the depth that anatomy understanding has within a yoga practice. Further exploration can uncover the relationship between physical anatomy and the energetic body, the connections between the physical body and the emotional body, and how the different layers interact with and impact each other. Prior to delving deeper into these topics, one must understand the basics.

With rates of participation in yoga skyrocketing and the type of people practicing yoga becoming more varied, the importance of safety and education among yoga teachers has never been higher. A well rounded education as a student, yoga teacher training, and continuing education pathway includes not only history and philosophy, energetics, emotional and subtle body, but must also include anatomy and physiology.

Thank you for making the investment in yourself as a student and/or teacher. By committing to deepening your understanding of anatomy and physiology you are playing a pivotal role in progressing the growth of yoga and the yoga industry.

Please be sure to visit www.livingwellwithlauren.com/critical-anatomy/ to stay up to date with locations and dates of upcoming in person anatomy trainings (which will enable you to teach anatomy to students and will provide you with 14 contact hours of Yoga Alliance certified continuing education) as well as information on upcoming books and learning materials.

Appendix A: The Student Manual

This manual creates an interactive approach to learning as well as a take home guide for yoga teacher trainees to use as a reference upon becoming teachers.

This manual may be reproduced for distribution to teacher trainees **only** by the teacher who purchased the Critical Anatomy book. All other distribution is strictly prohibited.

Systems of the Body:

- **Muscular**:_____

  _____

  _____

  _____

- **Skeletal**:_____

  _____

  _____

  _____

- **Nervous**:_____

  _____

  _____

  _____

- **Cardiovascular:**_____

  _____

  _____

  _____

- **Respiratory:**_____

  _____

  _____

  _____

- **Digestive:**_____

  _____

  _____

  _____

- **Endocrine:**_____

  _____

  _____

  _____

Muscular:

- There are approximately _____ skeletal muscles in the body.

- Anatomy of a muscle (draw below):

- Function of Muscles:

_____
_____
_____

- Connective Tissue:

_____
_____
_____
_____
_____

- Important muscles to know:

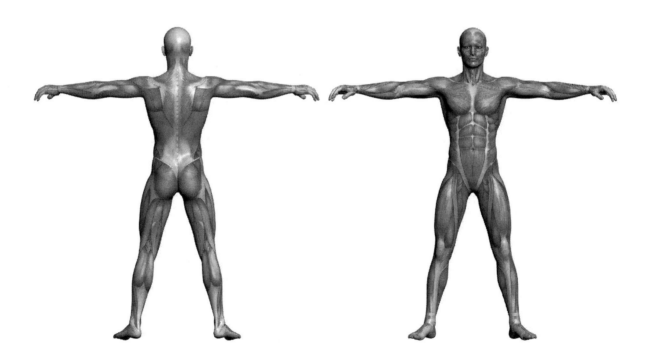

- Identify important musculature on the diagram. Use the area below to take notes on the muscles.

- The Back:

- The Abdominals:

- Posterior Hips:

- Hip Flexors:

- Quadriceps:

- Hamstrings:

- Upper Body:

Skeletal:

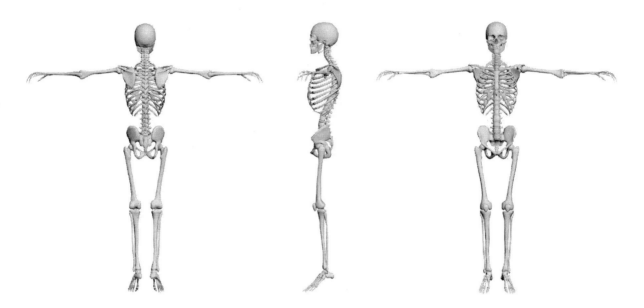

- There are ____ bones in the adult human body.
- Regions of the body:

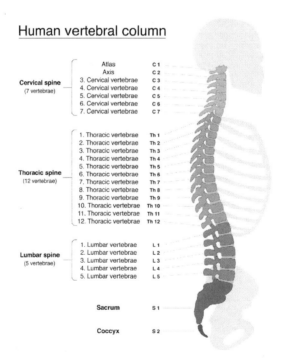

- Cervical spine: ___ vertebrae in neck.

    - C1: atlas. The joint between the occiput (skull) and C1 allows for

        _____.

- C2: axis. The joint between C1 and C2 allows for 50% of the _____ in the neck.
- All six motions are performed by the cervical spine (flexion, extension, rotation R/L, sidebending/lateral flexion R/L).

- Thoracic spine: ___ vertebrae in mid-back.

    - There is significantly less motion in the thoracic spine than in the cervical and lumbar spine, due to _____.

- Lumbar spine: ___ vertebrae in low back.

    - The most rotation in the lumbar spine occurs between _____.

- Pelvis:

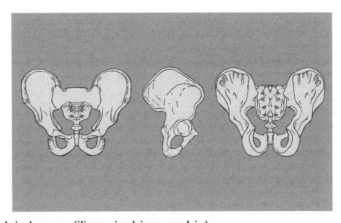

    - Pelvic bones (ilium, ischium, pubis):
        - The ischium are the "sitting bones" we refer to as yoga teachers.
    - Sacrum:
        - Very strongly associated with the movement of the low back, tilting of the sacrum facilitates movement of the lumbar spine.
    - Coccyx:
        - Tailbone.

    - Pelvic tilts:
        - Anterior:

        _____
        _____
        _____

        - Posterior:

_____
_____
_____

- We typically want:

_____
_____

- Ribcage:

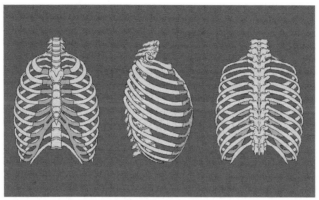

- True ribs: 1-7, attach directly to the sternum.
- False ribs: 8-10, share a cartilage attachment to the sternum.
- Floating ribs: 11-12, do not attach to sternum.
- Sternum: bony breastplate.
- Cuing:_____

_____
_____
_____

- Upper extremity:
    - Clavicle: the collarbone.
    - Scapula: the shoulder blade.
    - Humerus: the upper arm bone.
    - Radius/Ulna: bones of the forearm.
    - Carpals: wrist bones (8 of them).
    - Metacarpals: bones in the palm of the hand.
    - Phalanges: fingers.

- Lower extremity:
    - Femur: thigh bone.
    - Tibia/Fibula: bones of the lower leg.
    - Tarsals: ankle bones.
    - Metatarsals: foot bones.
    - Phalanges: toes.

- Types of joints and joint mechanics:

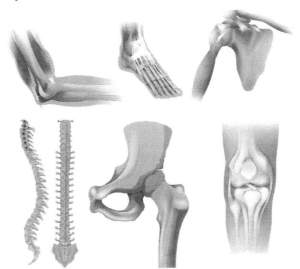

- Ball and socket:

_____
_____
_____
_____

- Hinge:

_____
_____
_____
_____

Nervous:

Human Nervous System (Male & Female)

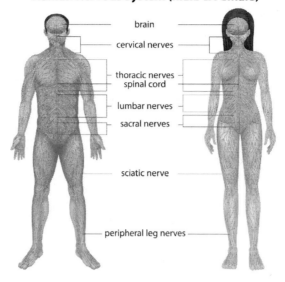

- The brain:

_____
_____
_____
_____
_____

- The spinal cord:

_____
_____
_____
_____

- Spinal nerves:

_____
_____
_____

  - Motor:

  _____
  _____
  _____

  - Sensory:

  _____

_____
_____

- Autonomic Nervous System:
    - Sympathetic:

        _____
        _____
        _____
        _____
        _____

    - Parasympathetic:

        _____
        _____
        _____
        _____
        _____

Cardiovascular:

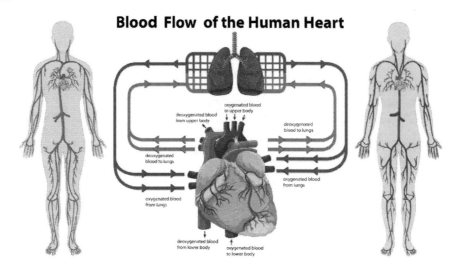

Blood Flow of the Human Heart

- The heart:

_____

_____

_____

_____

- Blood vessels:
    - Veins versus Arteries:

    _____

    _____

    _____

    _____

Respiratory:

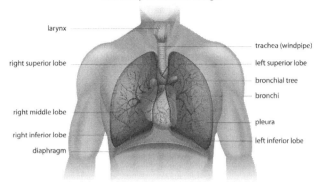

Anatomy of Human Lungs

larynx

trachea (windpipe)

right superior lobe

left superior lobe

bronchial tree

bronchi

right middle lobe

right inferior lobe

pleura

left inferior lobe

diaphragm

- The lungs:

_____

_____

_____

_____

- Mechanics of breathing:

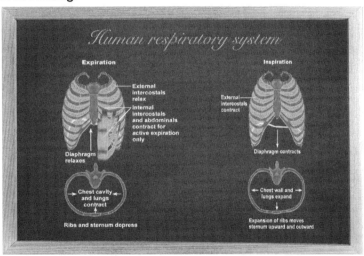

_____

_____

_____

_____

_____

Digestive System:

Human Digestive System

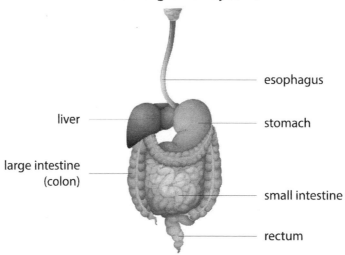

liver

esophagus

stomach

large intestine
(colon)

small intestine

rectum

- While the sympathetic nervous system is engaged and the body is in "fight or flight" mode, all of the blood:

_____

_____

- Yoga can change people to be more parasympathetic or "rest and digest" which results in:

_____

_____

- Postures for digestion:

_____

_____

_____

_____

_____

Endocrine System:

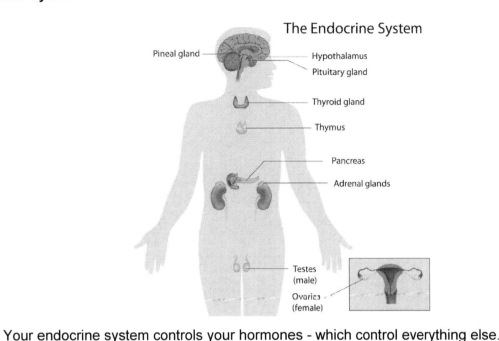

The Endocrine System

Pineal gland
Hypothalamus
Pituitary gland
Thyroid gland
Thymus
Pancreas
Adrenal glands
Testes (male)
Ovaries (female)

- Your endocrine system controls your hormones - which control everything else.
- Pituitary gland:

_____

_____

_____

- Thyroid and parathyroid:

_____

_____

_____

- Adrenals:

_____

_____

_____

- Pancreas:

_____

_____

_____

- Reproductive (ovaries/testicles):

_____

_____

_____

Common Yoga Injuries:

_____

_____

Neck:

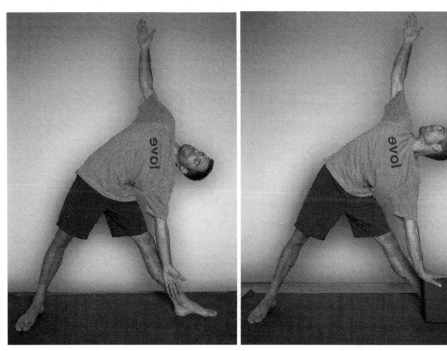

Triangle - Poor Cervical Alignment   Triangle - Correct Cervical Alignment

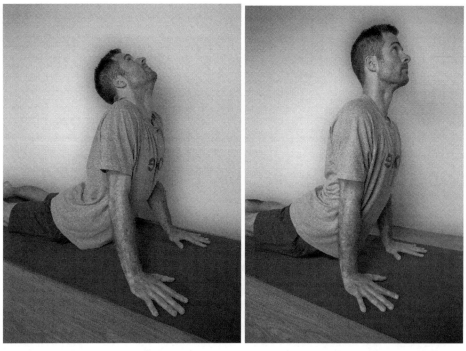

Upward Facing Dog - Poor Cervical Alignment   Upward Facing Dog - Correct Cervical Alignment

- Injuries:

_____
_____
_____
_____
_____

- Causes:

_____
_____
_____
_____
_____

- Prevention:

_____
_____
_____
_____
_____

- Modifications:

_____
_____
_____
_____
_____

Shoulder:

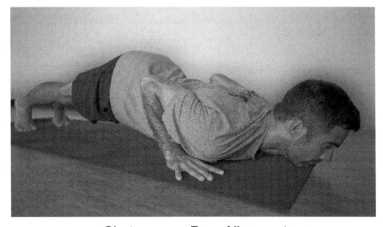

Chaturanga - Poor Alignment

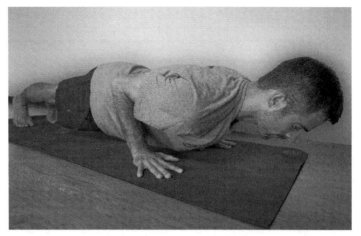

Chaturanga - Correct Alignment

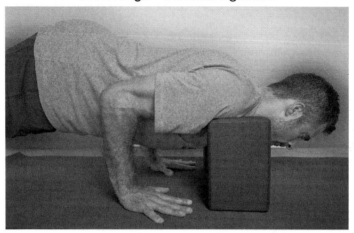

Chaturanga - Correct Alignment with Blocks

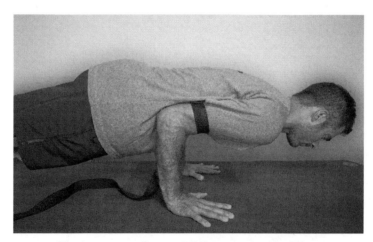

Chaturanga - Correct Alignment with Strap

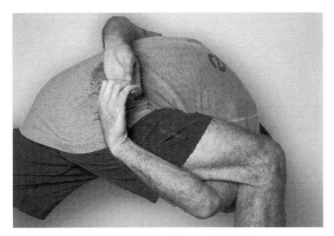

Bind - Incorrect, Posterior View

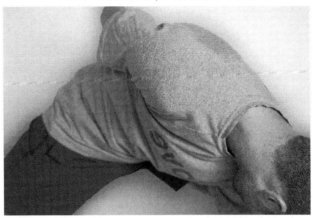

Bind - Incorrect, Anterior View

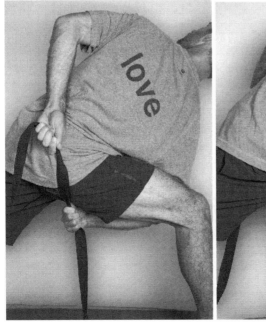
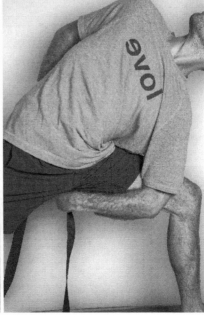

Bind - Correct, Posterior View   Bind - Correct, Anterior View

- Injuries:

  _____
  _____
  _____
  _____
  _____

- Causes:

  _____
  _____
  _____
  _____
  _____

- Prevention:

  _____
  _____
  _____
  _____
  _____

- Modifications:

  _____
  _____
  _____
  _____
  _____

Wrist:

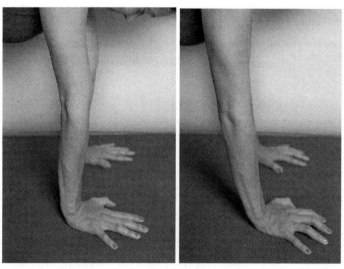

Elbow, Wrist, Hand Position - Incorrect   Elbow, Wrist, Hand Position - Correct

- Injuries:

_____
_____
_____
_____
_____

- Causes:

_____
_____
_____
_____
_____

- Prevention:

_____
_____
_____
_____
_____

- Modifications:

_____
_____
_____
_____
_____

Low Back:

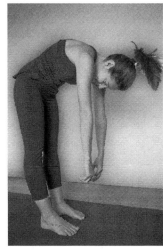 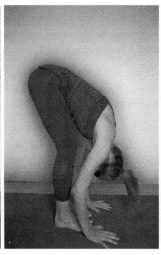 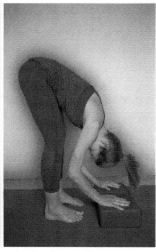

Forward Fold - Incorrect   Forward Fold - Correct   Forward Fold - Correct, with Blocks

- Injuries:

  _____
  _____
  _____
  _____
  _____

- Causes:

  _____
  _____
  _____
  _____
  _____

- Prevention:

  _____
  _____
  _____
  _____
  _____

- Modifications:

  _____
  _____
  _____
  _____
  _____

Knees:

- Injuries:

  _____
  _____
  _____
  _____
  _____

- Causes:

  _____
  _____
  _____
  _____
  _____

- Prevention:

_____

_____

_____

_____

_____

- Modifications:

_____

_____

_____

_____

_____

Best Ways to Prevent Yoga Injury:

- Understand anatomy and biomechanics!
- Clearly instruct students to listen to their own body. Each body is different, each pose will feel different to each person.
- Properly sequence classes for warm up, muscle and joint preparation, and safety.
    - Sequencing for backbends:
        - Muscles to activate:

        _____

        _____

        _____

        - Muscles to stretch:

        _____

        _____

        _____

        - Joints to open:

        _____

        _____

        _____

    - Sequencing for inversions:
        - Muscles to activate:

        _____

        _____

        _____

- Muscles to stretch:

  _____
  _____
  _____

- Joints to open:

  _____
  _____
  _____

- Sequencing for forward folds:
  - Muscles to activate:

    _____
    _____
    _____

  - Muscles to stretch:

    _____
    _____
    _____

  - Joints to open:

    _____
    _____
    _____

- Sequencing for arm balances:
  - Muscles to activate:

    _____
    _____
    _____

  - Muscles to stretch:

    _____
    _____
    _____

  - Joints to open:

    _____
    _____
    _____

  -

- Intently observe your students during class. Verbally or physically assist to correct students in postures that may cause injury.
- Take care with adjustments. Have an intention, be firm, sync with the student's breath, notice if the student seems uncomfortable.

What to do when a student has pain or is injured:
- Do not try to diagnose the problem. Know who to refer the student to, whether it's a physical therapist, chiropractor, or doctor, have people in the community you know and trust.
- Know the difference between pain and discomfort and what questions to ask to determine which the student is experiencing. Many people don't know the difference. Sharp, shooting, radiating, burning are all words that describe pain. Achy and dull indicate more of a discomfort feeling.
- Always encourage students not to push through pain (or significant discomfort) and to rest/avoid postures as needed.

Definitions and Concepts:

Stretching or Lengthening Muscles:
- To stretch or lengthen a muscle

  _____

  _____

- Different ways to stretch a muscle, safely and effectively:
  - "Stretch an active muscle":

    _____

    _____

    _____

    _____

  - Reciprocal inhibition:

    _____

    _____

    _____

    _____

- Stretching muscles that cross two joints:
  - Many muscles cross not one, but two joints. This makes stretching that muscle more complicated. You can stretch one end of it but stretching it at one joint, the other end of it by manipulating the other joint, or both ends of the muscle (the largest degree of stretch) by manipulating the positions of both joints.

Strengthening muscles:
- There are three types of contractions that cause strengthening of muscles.
    - Concentric contractions:

    _____
    _____
    _____

    - Eccentric contractions:

    _____
    _____
    _____

    - Isometric contractions:

    _____
    _____
    _____

    - Example: utkatasana (chair pose).

    _____
    _____
    _____

Joint mechanics:
- Certain patterns in different joints work together the best to result in the most motion with the least restriction. In yoga, the most important of these occur in the spine.
    - Cervical spine: when sidebending (lateral flexion), rotation to the _____ side occurs. Think of this when asking students to look in certain directions in poses.

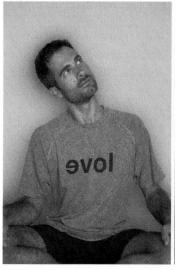
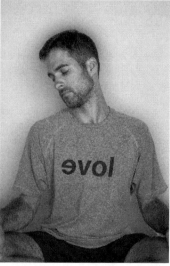

Cervical Rotation - Incorrect   Cervical Rotation - Correct

- Lumbar spine: when sidebending (lateral flexion), rotation to the _____ side occurs. Think of this when performing postures like utthita parsvakonasana.

- Capsular/closed packed position in shoulder:

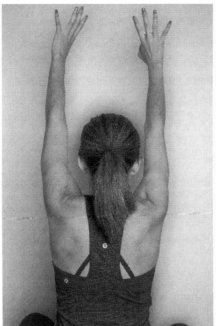 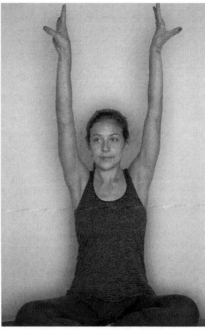

Overhead Reaching - Internal Rotation, Incorrect

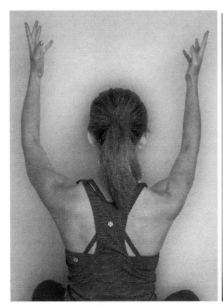 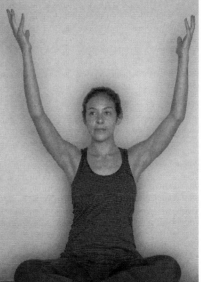

Overhead Reaching - External Rotation, Correct

_____

_____

Yoga Postures

Standing Postures:

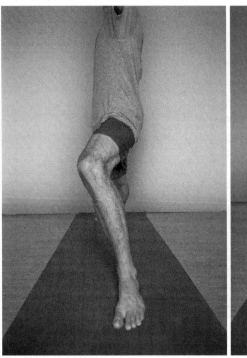 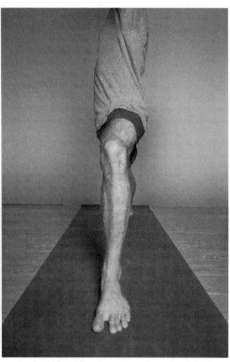

Warrior 2 - Incorrect Knee Alignment　　　　　Warrior 2 - Correct Knee Alignment

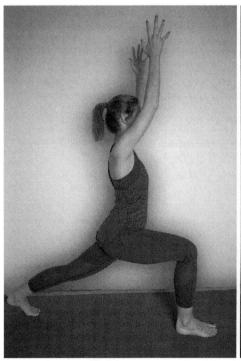 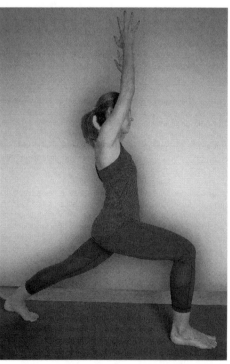

Crescent Lunge - Incorrect Lumbar and Shoulder Alignment　　Crescent Lunge - Correct Lumbar and Shoulder Alignment

- General muscle groups involved:

_____

_____

_____

_____

- Joints/alignment:

_____

_____

_____

_____

- Important biomechanics:

_____

_____

_____

_____

- Example poses:

_____

_____

_____

_____

Balance Postures:

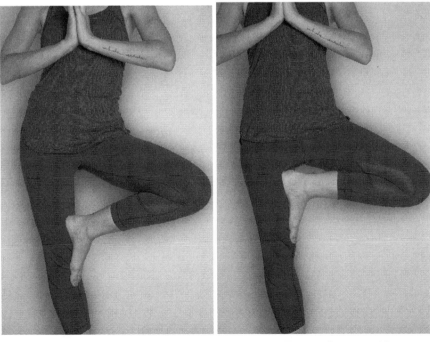

Tree - Incorrect Alignment   Tree - Correct Alignment

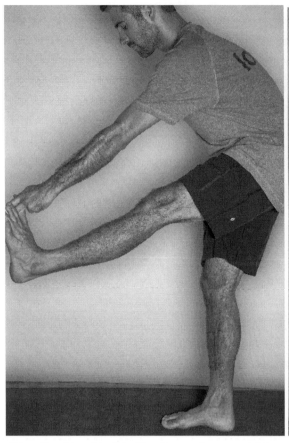 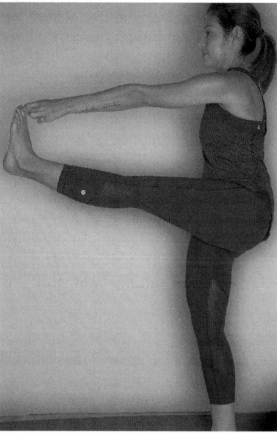

Standing Hand to Big Toe Pose - Incorrect Alignment   Standing Hand to Big Toe Pose - Correct Alignment

- General muscle groups involved:

_____

_____

_____

_____

- Joints/alignment:

_____

_____

_____

_____

- Important biomechanics:

_____

_____

_____

_____

- Example poses:

_____

_____

_____

_____

Backbends:

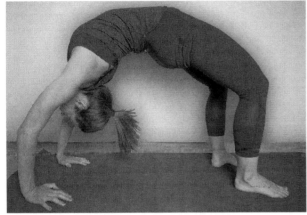 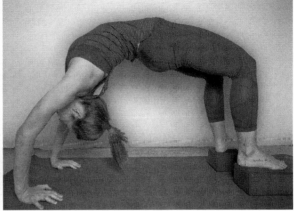

Wheel - Improper Alignment (hinge)   Wheel - Proper Alignment, with Blocks

- General muscle groups involved:

_____

_____

_____

_____

- Joints/alignment:

_____

_____

_____

_____

- Important biomechanics:

_____

_____

_____

_____

- Example poses:

_____

_____

Forward Bends:

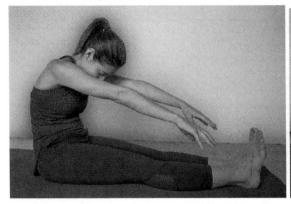
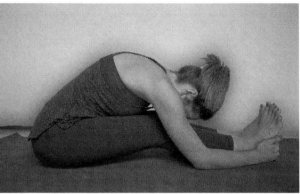

Seated Forward Fold - Incorrect Alignment   Seated Forward Fold - Correct Alignment

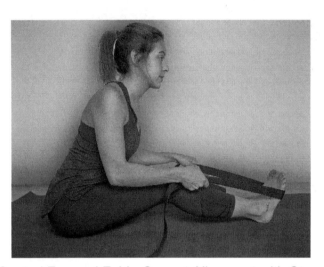

Seated Forward Fold - Correct Alignment with Strap

- General muscle groups involved:

_____

_____

_____

_____

- Joints/alignment:

_____

_____

_____

_____

-   Important biomechanics:

_____

_____

_____

_____

-   Example poses:

_____

_____

_____

_____

Twists:

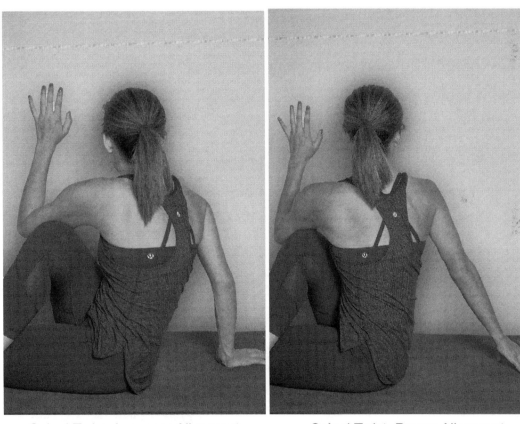

Spinal Twist- Improper Alignment   Spinal Twist- Proper Alignment

-   General muscle groups involved:

_____

_____

_____

_____

- Joints/alignment:

- Important biomechanics:

- Example poses:

Inversions:

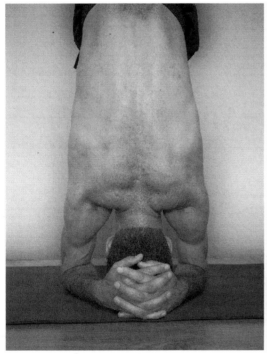 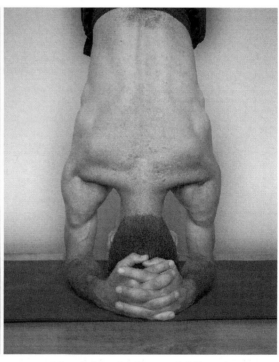

Headstand - Incorrect Alignment   Headstand - Correct Alignment

- General muscle groups involved:

_____
_____

- Joints/alignment:

_____
_____
_____
_____

- Important biomechanics:

_____
_____
_____
_____

- Example poses:

_____
_____
_____
_____

Arm Balances:

- General muscle groups involved:

_____
_____
_____
_____

- Joints/alignment:

_____
_____
_____
_____

- Important biomechanics:

_____
_____
_____
_____

- Example poses:

_____
_____

_____
_____

Hip Openers:
-   General muscle groups involved:

_____
_____
_____
_____

-   Joints/alignment:

_____
_____
_____
_____

-   Important biomechanics:

_____
_____
_____
_____

-   Example poses:

_____
_____
_____
_____

Competency Quiz

1. When teachers instruct students to "tuck their tailbone" they are encouraging which type of pelvic tilt, anterior or posterior?
2. What are some poses that might be uncomfortable for students based on their hip anatomy?
3. True or false: In an open hip posture, the hips face the same direction as the shoulders.
4. Is upward facing dog an appropriate warm up for backbending?
5. True or false: The cervical spine likes to rotate and sidebend in opposite directions.
6. The most injured joint in yoga is _____.
7. Name two reasons for giving a student an adjustment in a pose.
8. True or false: The diaphragm contracts during exhalation.
9. Name the most important muscle of the anterior core.
10. The "master gland" is the _____ gland.

Made in the USA
San Bernardino, CA
10 October 2017